THE WOMAN'S HOUR BOOK

THE WOMAN'S HOUR BOOK

**Edited by Wyn Knowles
and Kay Evans**

INTRODUCED BY SUE MACGREGOR

Illustrations by Phillida Gili

SIDGWICK & JACKSON . LONDON
BRITISH BROADCASTING CORPORATION

First published in Great Britain by Sidgwick & Jackson Limited
and the British Broadcasting Corporation in 1981

© British Broadcasting Corporation and Contributors 1981
Illustrations © Phillida Gili 1981

Sidgwick & Jackson ISBN 0-283-98821-5
BBC ISBN 0-563-20013-8

Printed in Great Britain by
Biddles Ltd, Guildford, Surrey
for Sidgwick & Jackson Limited
1 Tavistock Chambers, Bloomsbury Way
London WC1A 2SG
and the British Broadcasting Corporation
35 Marylebone High Street
London W1M 4AA

INTRODUCTION

Sue MacGregor

Woman's Hour is something of a BBC institution, which could make us feel dangerously smug. It has been going with barely an interruption for thirty-five years, and though from time to time over the years its skirtlength may have been hoicked up or let down, and its waistline hitched in or expanded, the whole outfit is still recognizably cut from the same pattern of those post-war New Look days of 1946 when the first programme went out, though thank heavens the cloth itself gets constantly renewed. Extraordinarily enough, *Woman's Hour* was first presented by a man. Did the BBC really feel that the views of 'an ordinary housewife' and an interview with budding actress Deborah Kerr, which were indeed part of the very first edition, would be more acceptable to fledgeling listeners if a chap was in charge? Since then, almost without exception, a woman's voice has introduced and greeted; professional broadcasters like Judith Chalmers, Jean Metcalfe and for many years Marjorie Anderson have compèred what Russell Harty once called 'The Hour'. In those days he was a lowly producer of book programmes along the corridor, and could be persuaded to impersonate 'a mere male from Worthing' in our listeners' letters column.

It is nine years since I became part of the *Woman's Hour* team. I wasn't at all sure then what I had let myself in for, as I came straight from *The World at One* and *PM*, which meant that when *Woman's Hour* was on the air I was both recovering from one deadline and preparing to meet another. Now, however, it seems so much a part of my life that I have found myself in absent-minded moments at home snatching up the telephone and announcing to startled friends that they have reached *Woman's Hour*.

How, people often ask, is the programme created? Is it 'live'? How many of you work on it? Some people have the extraordinary impression that it all happens by some miraculous process of spontaneous combustion at two minutes past two, precisely. It is rather more complicated than that, of course, and if the general impression we give on the air is one of calm and control, it is all the result of a great deal of discussion, argument, and ideas; endless hours of recording and editing tape; persuading some

5

speakers, discouraging others; disagreement, cross-pollination, and above all fun – sometimes quite noisy fun. The team numbers approximately ten: the editor, Wyn Knowles, her deputy, Kay Evans, and around eight producers, among whose number at the last count were two men. But within the team producers still have their own specialities: rather to my amazement I see on the current list that someone has marine biology close to her heart. Producers usually work away at their own pieces of the programme well ahead of time – sometimes months ahead. They also take it in turn to produce the daily edition, making sure that it hangs together as a whole and fits into the rigid time slot. Incidentally, someone should report us for contravening the Trades Descriptions Act. We no longer last an hour; for some time now we have been reduced to just under fifty-eight minutes.

It could be a relentless treadmill, doing four programmes a week from London, so the fifth, on Friday, comes from one of the BBC's regions to ensure that the metropolis doesn't hog it all. Our Tuesday morning phone-in and our Sunday edition, *Weekend*, complete the list.

Everyone has a shrewd idea of the contents of each day's programme several days in advance, although the truly 'live' parts are to a certain extent unknown quantities. For instance, twice a week we have a 'live' discussion on something topical: it could be on opinion polls and how they are conducted, or the current situation in Poland, or on what it's like to give birth to a handicapped child, or even on something potentially very tricky like incest. One of our producers will have chosen the topic and the speakers, and we will all have done our homework, but even though we all meet up in advance over sandwiches and coffee (in the lavish old days it was a three-course lunch, I'm told; austerity has struck), the temperature of what looks like a good idea on paper can only truly be tested in the studio after the green light has flashed to tell us we're 'on'. Speakers can be nervous and dry up, or talk too fast; they can arrive late and harassed; they can be too confident in advance – a fatal mistake. Mostly, however, they rise splendidly to the challenge. So do our special guests, who have a fifteen-minute slot to themselves in the Wednesday programme, also 'live'. The beneficial powers of the quick flow of adrenalin that 'live' performance needs are not to be sneezed at, though poor Sebastian Coe almost needed a tranquilliser when a

6

taxi took him for a tour of Wandsworth before dropping him at Broadcasting House only minutes before he was due on. If we both sounded a little short of breath that day, it was not because he had taken me on a quick training run up Portland Place!

Other parts of the programme, such as complicated features, interviews done away from base, book reviews and the serial reading, are recorded, and the tapes played in round my linking remarks. These tapes, by the way, may have taken many days' advance work to prepare: one ten-minute feature on, say, living in a new town, may be the result of three days' work from the reporter and many hours of producers' editing and discussion before it is finally put together in a studio ready for broadcast.

The programme is relayed from a studio deep underground. If you think you hear a faint rumbling from time to time, it's the Bakerloo Line operating not many yards away. The people who put out each day's programme – producer, technical operators, presenter, 'live' guests and their producers – descend mole-like to this studio in relays. We don't rehearse the programme, as they used to in the old days, so that the 'live' transmission between two and three o'clock will be our first opportunity to find out whether it all works as it should.

Afterwards, there is discussion and criticism, and then preparation for the next day's edition, usually within half an hour of the conclusion of the current one. And because what we do one day has disappeared into the ether the next – unless some sympathetic archivist has her preserving kit handy – it's nice to have, from time to time, a reminder of some parts of *Woman's Hour* which we have enjoyed preparing and listening to ourselves over the past year or so. This is what you will find on the pages that follow.

S.M.

Some of the pieces have been transcribed from interviews by Ron Alldridge, Annie Allsebrook, Gill Cochrane, Kay Evans, Jane Finnis, Judy Graham, David Hawksworth, Anne Howells, Helen Lloyd, Sue MacGregor, Pat McLoughlin, Margaret Percy, Pat Rowe, Diana Stenson, David Williams and Joan Yorke.

SPRING

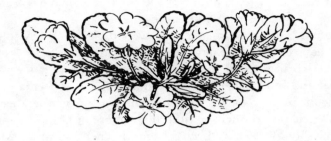

COUNTRY DIARY

*Robin Page on the countryside in March**

The grass is now becoming greener, the birds are singing louder and a feeling of spring and regeneration is in the air. Many people have their own particular signs of spring that they look for, and my favourite is the colour-change in starlings' beaks. In winter they are dark and drab, but now they are a vivid yellow, almost primrose colour. If you look at the starlings in your garden they will all have these beautifully coloured beaks.

Most people think starlings are dull and drab, but in fact they are attractive birds. Their plumage is iridescent in sunlight and you see flashes of mauve, blue and turquoise. They are also very amusing birds, too; on several days I went out of the farmhouse and thought I could hear a curlew, but it was only a starling sitting in a tree mimicking. One day I also thought I could hear my father whistling our disobedient border collie dog from the top of a weeping willow tree, which was very strange. But again it was a starling that had picked up this distinctive whistle and was thoroughly enjoying himself.

One evening thousands and thousands of starlings came over in great waves. It's known as a pre-roost flight, and they gather together in a vast mass before going to their dusk roosting place. It was an amazing sight. Some people say they spread foot and mouth disease, and March was a worrying time, because we let our beef cattle and our one remaining dairy cow out on the grass this month and of course they mix with starlings.** The animals, dancing and gambolling, were pleased to get out from their winter confinement. When we changed the time they danced and gambolled by getting out of the field at four o'clock in the morning, which was rather appalling.

Other birds that gave me pleasure were rooks. A nearby spinney used to have twenty-four nests; then last year a farmer set a crow-scarer which frightened them all away. But this year they have returned and built seventeen nests. Alas, there has been a 40 per cent decline in the rook population in the last thirty years, because of the destruction of their habitat and the use of pesticide sprays.

March should also have been the month when I saw mad March hares, but I only saw one. The reason for their scarcity is again said to be sprays – Gramoxone, which is used on a lot of crops. When the hares lick themselves they swallow the poison. Although this has been going on for several years no research has been done, and the hare population has plummeted.

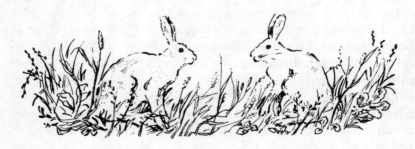

It should also have been a time for seeing frogs and frogspawn. When I was a child, just after the Second World War, we had a pond near our brook which always had bucketfuls of spawn in it. In fact as the water level dropped I would transfer literally buckets and buckets of frogspawn into the brook itself to stop the tadpoles from drying up. I went to all the old sites, but found no spawn at all and no sign of a frog. And since the river authority has cleaned the brook, so that the water rushes down it, even if the frogs do spawn it all gets washed away. It is a sad aspect of the countryside that the frog, a creature involved in folklore and folk medicine and all sorts of other things, is just disappearing. The Wildlife and Countryside Bill is thirty years too late – at least it's much too late for the common frog.

But there were some good things still. The spring flowers were particularly pleasant – daffodils and primroses in the garden, and in the hedgerows violets, pussy willow, lesser celandine and colts-foot. The yellow coltsfoot flower comes first, followed by the leaf, which, as the name suggests, is shaped like a colt's foot. I always think it is interesting how old country names, such as pheasant's eye and ox tongue, link flowers with animals and birds.

* A full account of life throughout the year on the Pages' Cambridgeshire farm can be read in *The Journal of a Country Parish*, published by Davis-Poynter

**There was an outbreak of foot-and-mouth disease on the Isle of Wight at the time of this broadcast

WEDDING DAY MEMORIES

Three people describe their varied wedding day experiences. First Ba Mason recalls her wartime wedding and its combination of austerity and elegance

On the dawn of my great day I realized with dismay that I was feeling rather ill. I had spent the previous evening sitting in the cellar, a million curlers wound in my hair, while buzz-bombs chugged monotonously and lethally over London. Still, I'd spent many a night in the same circumstances without feeling any ill-effects. When at last the All Clear sounded and we stumbled upstairs I'd stopped worrying whether my husband-to-be – who was, I know, idling away the hours in a night club – would change his mind and leave me at the church. All I cared about was getting my aching head on my pillow.

I awoke to find our doctor by my bed, counting my pulse and observing me closely. I felt I must be seriously ill to warrant such an early call on her part. As I opened my eyes she tipped a white powder on my tongue and pattered rapidly away. I heard her call out to my mother, 'She'll do.' I began to feel perfectly well and got up and went downstairs. The house was bursting with people and all of them appeared too busy to spare a word to the heroine of the hour. My father had withdrawn to some inaccessible hiding-place and was peacefully smoking his after-breakfast pipe and reading the paper.

Suddenly, my mother swooped down and told me it was high

time I got dressed. In front of the long mirror in her room I regarded myself arrayed in my wedding dress, which was constructed from un-couponed Nottingham lace curtain material. I wasn't enthralled by my reflection. Then a friend of my mother's burst into my privacy and, snatching my tulle veil, crushed it down on my head as far as my eyebrows in the manner of the present Queen Mother when she married the future King George VI. I wore my hair then in a fringe, copied from a film star I admired called Paulette Goddard. My fiancé had made it clear that he didn't care for my fringe; like his new moustache, which I didn't much go for either, it was an innovation acquired since the days when we had first met. I lied to him – I told him my wedding veil and head-dress had been specially designed to wear with a fringe. Actually, it had been lent to me. As arranged by Mummy's bossy friend, I looked like a commando with a mass of leaves and twigs and orange blossoms camouflaging his helmet.

Furiously I yanked it back and stamped downstairs, where my father, winkled out, was waiting to conduct me to the church in a black, hearse-like hired car. The February weather was ghastly and Daddy chose to wear a very old Harris tweed overcoat over his finery. I, in white lace curtaining, was expected to brave the elements. At the church a verger knelt reverently to spread out my long tulle veil. Daddy appeared to have no intention of removing his awful coat. The organist stopped twiddling and footling about and burst into my entry music, Elgar's *Enigma Variations*. The doors were thrown open. I'd either have to go up the aisle alone, or with a father in Harris tweed. Suddenly he wrestled himself out of it, grabbed my arm and said, unforgivably, 'Stop dithering about.'

I remember well how astonished I was that none of my friends and relations on the left of the church gave us so much as a smile. They stood and stared like a lot of suspicious bullocks when a dog enters their field. I saw with relief not one, but two, uniformed figures waiting at the altar. For a mad moment I wondered if I was going to be duelled over; then sanity returned and I recognized the best man. As I knelt to be joined in holy matrimony I was acutely aware that my last pair of nylons had laddered from ankle to knee.

I enjoyed our reception so much that I had to be told three times, with increasing sternness, that it was time to leave. I came down the stairs in my utility suit and hurled away my bouquet, which was caught with a screech of joy by our Irish maid who was three months pregnant by a wandering GI.

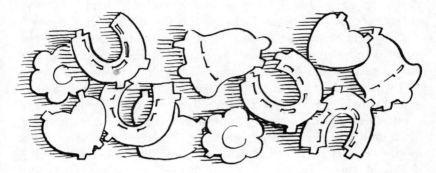

We spent the first night of the honeymoon at the Savoy. I changed into what was known as a little black dress and we went down to the bar where my husband bought an evening paper and read it with concentrated attention. It had been a long day and I was reasonably content to sit in silence watching the people. One of my officers walked by. I was working in MI5 at the time, in a department which has recently come in for a lot of publicity. In the euphoria of being on honeymoon I called out to him and waved. He passed me silently, with a surly expression. I'd forgotten for a second that I worked for the secret service.

In the middle of the ensuing night I dreamed vividly about Fred MacMurray, a film actor I particularly disliked, and woke, screaming: 'I never thought it would be like this. . . .' My brother had said it would be a miracle if any man ever married me, but I think it's a miracle I wasn't divorced then and there.

Writer and journalist Hunter Davies with recollections of his wedding to fellow-writer and reviewer Margaret Forster

We were married on 11 June 1960, which I remember very well as I was there at the time. My wife, who was with me, was still technically a student, and had got special permission to get married a few days before the end of term. We were married at Oxford Register Office, which didn't please our parents – in fact, not much about our wedding day did please our parents. We'd only been going out for centuries, as we'd grown up together in Carlisle, but they seemed to look upon it as some sort of surprise.

I drove down from London in my very first car, a 1947 2.5 litre Riley, which I had bought for £100, and in which I'd failed my driving test three times. I was working at the time on a newspaper, now deceased, called the *Sunday Graphic*, and I felt very pleased with myself, having got on to a London newspaper after only nine months in journalism. I used to wear my green eyeshade all the time. Perhaps that's why I kept on failing my driving test.

I wore my best and only suit, a sort of sharp Italian job, all the rage, which I'd bought the previous year in Manchester; I couldn't afford a new one. I kept on pulling it down at the back because it was one of those suits with very, very short jackets – a bum-freezer, I think it was called. Now what did my wife wear? I should know, because I've seen the photographs. Something white, I think.

Afterwards we drove out to the Bear at Woodstock, where I told everyone they could have anything they liked for lunch, though I carefully ordered the cheapest items for myself, having seen the prices on the menu. Then we sent special cards to our parents, telling them we'd just got married. We thought this was very witty, but they didn't think it was at all amusing.

We drove back to London in the evening to our first home, a flat in the Vale of Health in Hampstead. I'd been living there alone for a few weeks, and I'd stocked the fridge with bacon and kippers for breakfast the next morning, when we were due to fly out to Sardinia for our honeymoon. The smell was terrible when we got into the flat – I'd forgotten all about the kippers. She refused to eat them, and said she hated fried bacon, and why had I bought them, and how stupid – anyway, that was our first row. I ate all the kippers and bacon on my own. All the way to the airport I felt terribly sick.

Our parents approved of our marriage – I don't want to suggest they were against it – but it was just that they would have liked a church service and a big do afterwards. We just wanted to be alone. But if *my* children sneak off and do *me* out of a big family party, I'll be furious!

My best friend and I were having a supportive gin and tonic as we got me ready. It was a cold, sunny day in January, and instead of doing the shopping and going to the pub I was going off to be married. So many of the family and friends had come over from Ireland that I was able to get them group reductions and arrange a deal with the airline and hotel. Although in my thirties, I was as excited as any teenager, and just as full of nerves.

One of the anxieties was the best man, who was organizing the transport to the register office. He is one of those people who always arrive for trains with ten seconds to spare, whereas I am one of those people who arrive half an hour early. Was there any real danger, I wondered, that he would leave it too late, and we'd get caught up in traffic and miss our wedding? But a whole hour before I expected him, he arrived – with the groom – and announced that the time had come.

'They're really overdoing it this time', I said, full of anxiety again in case he had some plan for us to fill in the spare hour by going to the Tower of London or on a cruise up the Thames.

From our various robing rooms, adjusting ties and straightening hats, we converged at the front gate demanding to know why we were being given such a great margin of safety. And then we saw them! Two gigantic horses, a huge carriage, two footmen in uniform, with fur rugs and a bottle of champagne . . . all waiting to take us to our wedding. Now I am known to be the sort of person who enjoys showing off, but never in my wildest dreams could I have thought up something like this. The man I married is a gentle person, not an extrovert, and in his headiest fantasy he could not have come up with anything so outrageous.

We settled in and clopped off to Hammersmith, to the amazement of everyone in West London. Near Hammersmith roundabout we worried in case the horses couldn't cope with the traffic, but not a bit of it. They were used to being in films like *Ben Hur*, and obviously they thought this was dead easy. I later learned that, while the family and friends were waiting for us at the register office, somebody had asked my sister, 'Are you with the coach and horses party?'

'Aren't the English extraordinary?' my sister had thought.

15

'Imagine having a coach and horses!' Then we came round the corner.

The sun shone and the buses hooted, and passers-by waved, and as we trotted off to the reception afterwards we got a taste of what it's like being famous. In fact we'd developed quite a gracious and, dare I say it, even elegant, way of greeting the stunned crowds, who assumed we must be part of a very unusual film, or minor foreign royalty. What we didn't anticipate was how quickly we would grow to like it, and to feel that we wouldn't mind travelling around like that all the time. It was a very good start to our married life. As we both said, when we first saw the horses, 'If we can go through with this, we can go through with anything!'

CHINESE GHOST WEDDINGS

Frena Bloomfield

I have always found weddings rather a chore, but I was invited to one in Hong Kong that was quite unusual. For a start, the two main characters were dead. The bride and bridegroom had both died years before as small children; they had never known each other in life, and their families had come together only for this rather special occasion. It was a ghost wedding.

Ghost weddings aren't common in Hong Kong, but probably a couple of hundred are still carried out every year. I heard about one that took place in a Chinese friend's family. Her mother had a dream in which a young man appeared who identified himself as her son who had died in infancy. He had met a young woman in the ghost world, he said, her name was so-and-so, her family still lived at such-and-such address, and he wanted a ghost marriage arranged. When his mother woke up she recalled the dream very clearly. Saying nothing to anyone else, she went to the address he had mentioned in the dream. There she found a family of the name given: they had indeed had a daughter who had died as a child, and her name was the one stated by the woman's son in the dream.

This is typical of the way in which such marriages often start,

16

and frankly there's no way to explain it. It just happens. It's more rare for the marriages to be arranged at the initiation of the families, but that does also happen. If they want to marry off a dead child, they will go either to a Taoist priest or to a woman spirit medium, of which there are still quite a number in Hong Kong.

Most Westerners, of course, would query why anyone would want to marry the dead to each other and, indeed, as far as I know, though I'm not an anthropologist, the Chinese are unique in doing this. For those who believe in it, it does serve a purpose. It tidies up the family tree, leaving no loose ends. It also keeps the dead happy, or so their families feel, and this will guarantee that the spirits of the dead don't come back to cause trouble for the living. Those who do accept it find nothing remarkable in the practice. When I asked a woman spirit medium why the dead wanted to marry, she looked rather astonished and said: 'But they'd be lonely otherwise.'

Surprisingly, this kind of event occurs at all levels of society, from rich and sophisticated urbanites down to poor farmers in rural areas. Sometimes the marriage is carried out for social reasons – an older son, although dead, should still be married before a younger one, so his parents might marry him off once the younger, living son wants to get married.

The wedding I attended was held in a tiny back street flat, two floors up in a rather squalid building. Street noises came in at the open balcony and we could hear kids playing outside. The very elderly parents of the dead children came along, but no one else. It's not quite like a live wedding, where the whole family comes. There were wedding presents, however – a double bed, a television, some jewellery, and household objects even down to a thermos flask and mugs. The only odd note is that all these things are always made of paper; later they're burned and their essence is transferred to the underworld. A large, ornate paper couple represent the bride and groom, and they are attended by paper gods and goddesses, guardians of the underworld. After a long ritual before a large altar, the woman medium pronounced the couple married, and everything and everybody was burned up in an incinerator in the corner. The parents of the bride and groom left together after the ceremony to have a celebration meal and afterwards, presumably, they went their separate ways.

Sometimes, however, families really do unite through the weddings. Each child will be written into the other's family scroll, and living family members on both sides will make offerings for them. Very rarely the family may actually adopt a living child on behalf of the ghost couple. It's an odd custom, but it underlines the strength of the Chinese family structure – even if you're dead, they still try to look after you.

CHASING THE DRAGON

*Jackie Pullinger, a committed Christian, talks about her experiences while running a youth club in a slum area in Hong Kong**

When I first set up the club I wasn't sure what to expect. I knew there were many drug addicts, but I didn't feel scared – in fact quite the reverse, a rather extraordinary, illogical joy. I actually enjoyed being there, and I began to get to know some of the people. I found boys who had run away from home when they were five or six, and others who didn't have the opportunity to go to school and just wanted to get work on a noodle stall in the street. They slept in gang pads and even in the street, and were drawn into gang activities at a very young age indeed. I very much wanted to reach these boys.

We had a certain amount of difficulty with the Triads, though to start with we had some nice people in the youth club, and that was because they thought I was a nice person, and they had the idea that missionaries were there to help them as under-privileged people. What they wanted was an introduction to a job or a school. 'Can you get me to America?' they would ask, or 'Can you get my family free rice?' It wasn't for about three years that they realized I had no money, because I had no official church backing. Then I lost all the nice ones and all the nasty ones remained – the real street kids and the thugs. They were there because I liked them and they liked me. 'Well, of course, she's cracked about Jesus,' they said, 'but apart from that she's all right.'

I never tried to persuade anyone to become a Christian, and I never told anyone not to take drugs – it would have been a complete waste of time. But after a few years one of the boys said to me:

'Why are you still here? We kick you. We take you for every penny you've got. You send us to school and we don't go. You find us homes and we muck them up. You find us jobs and we don't go. Why do you stay around?'

I replied that Jesus loved me, and that he loved my questioner too.

'Well,' the young man said, 'he couldn't love people like us, because we rape people.' It's true – they do this professionally. They get girls into trouble and then sell them; it's a form of income. 'We have to fight and steal', he went on. 'Nobody would love us like that.'

I replied that I knew it was very unfair that Jesus should love him since he was like that, but nevertheless he did. I told the young man in a very simple way that all the awful things he said he did, Jesus had in fact said that he himself did, and that if the young man were to give them all to Jesus, Jesus would give him his nice, clean life back.

He was so shattered that he just sat down in the street and said, 'Well, Jesus, if you really are God, please change me.'

He was my first converted Triad, and it certainly wasn't the result of any persuasion from me – he was just so amazed that anybody should love him in that way. After that event he used to bring back his friends every week, and we went higher and higher up their hierarchy, because everybody has a kind of 'big brother'. They all used to bring one along, and we found we were really working through this particular Triad society.

The prostitutes presented a very difficult problem. Some of the girls I first knew were twelve or so and had been sold into prostitution. I couldn't even talk to them because they were virtually prisoners, guarded by old women. But there was one particular group I used to pass as I went into the club every night – they were all drug addicts as well, of course, and had scar marks on the backs of their hands. I'd been going in and out for years saying in Chinese, 'Jesus loves you', and they would all nod and smile but of course it didn't mean anything very much. After a few years, when we had brought a large number of the Triad boys off drugs – and they came off quite painlessly, without withdrawal symptoms, when they became Christians – it occurred to me I couldn't actually tell any of the girls about Jesus, because if they believed, I had nowhere to put them. Clearly you can't put prostitutes in your house with young boys, even if they do want to be Christians, so I rather avoided telling them.

One day, however, I couldn't resist the opportunity. There was a really pathetic one called Ah Ping who had nowhere to live. The only way she got a bed was if a man hired her, and then she would spend the night at whatever place he had paid for. I told her a little bit about Jesus, and I didn't get through, so then I told her the story about the prostitute who washed Jesus' feet with her hair. Ah Ping's eyes lit up and she said, 'That's the one! That's the God I want to believe in – the one that loved the prostitute.'

I said that he could change her life, and that it was very simple if she would just ask him to. So she sat on an orange box in the street and began to pray. Her pimp, an old coolie, was splitting his sides because he thought it was so funny, but she wasn't daunted. She just sat there praying quite happily, and I prayed with her. After about five minutes I thought we had done enough, but she went on praying and began to praise God in a new language which she had never learned – which is what happened to the disciples when they were filled with God's Holy Spirit.

At the end she looked up, radiant with happiness, and I suddenly wondered what I was going to do with her. On that particular day I had no money at all on me, and there was nowhere for her to go – nobody wants a just-converted prostitute to sleep on their floor. So I had to say, 'I'm terribly sorry, but I'm going to have to leave you here.' She sat on her orange box, looking around for the men, so then I added, 'Now that you're going to follow Jesus, you don't actually have to look to men any more for your living.' But even as I was saying it I wondered how she was going to get her food and rent money.

'Well, is my rice going to fall down from heaven?' she inquired.

I answered that I supposed it might, since God could do that.

She caught hold of this idea, and said, 'Tell you what – next time I see you, I'll let you know how it comes.'

I never saw Ah Ping there again, and when I asked her friends where she was they said she had gone away somewhere to get off drugs, and that she wasn't a prostitute any more. I never found out where she had gone, but I really do believe that she changed, and God did find a place for her to live and means for her to live on.

*Her book on the subject, *Chasing the Dragon*, is published by Hodder and Stoughton

COOKING IN A WOK

Cookery writer Marika Hanbury Tenison on an unusual, ancient, but very clever piece of kitchen equipment

The wok is one of the best things that ever happened to cookery. It's a Chinese frying pan, invented many thousands of years ago because the Chinese had two problems: food was very expensive, and so was fuel. So they developed a pan that would cook quickly and cheaply, and in which you could cook finely chopped ingredients, combining vegetables with a small amount of more expensive meat, poultry or fish to produce nourishing but inexpensive dishes. It doesn't have a flat bottom like other pans. In fact it's like a very wide, shallow bowl, and the shape means that the whole surface heats up very quickly. It's made of very thin metal, which also assists speedy heating. So really it takes no time at all to cook food in a wok.

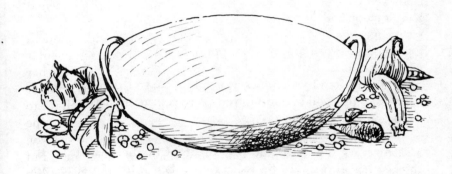

Some woks have a little collar, a useful device if you're going to use an electric plate, because it keeps the wok steady and stops it rolling around. I use a camping stove for my wok, though, because it's got a good flame and is very cheap to run – it's much cheaper than electricity, for instance. It's also marvellous if you go camping, because you can fry eggs, casserole, steam, stew – in fact you can do anything in a wok. My husband Robin is an explorer, and when I accompanied him on one jungle expedition, cooking for forty-five people every day, I found that a wok was the only utensil fast enough and economical enough for my requirements. I learned to use two woks, frying rice in one, and vegetables and meat in the other.

This is a delicious, economical dish which will feed six people even though it uses only one chicken leg. Another advantage of this sort of cooking is that you can do your preparation in advance. All the vegetables can be prepared and chopped or sliced the night before. That's why woks are such a marvellous boon for people who are out at work all day. Put your prepared vegetables in covered polythene boxes, then when you get home it will take you about 6 to 8 minutes to cook them, and 20 minutes to cook the rice.

Marinade (prepare the day before)
1 tablespoon cornflour
1 tablespoon soft brown sugar
1 tablespoon soy sauce
1 tablespoon dry sherry or any other available alcohol (optional)

Other ingredients
1 chicken leg
2 tablespoons oil
1 clove garlic
1 piece fresh green ginger ⎫
1 green chilli ⎬ optional
⎭
small quantities of vegetables as available, e.g. 1 onion, 1 carrot, sprigs of broccoli or cauliflower, peas, courgettes, lettuce
1 chicken stock cube

Mix together the marinade ingredients. Cut the meat from the chicken leg into small, thin slices and then into thin strips and place them in the marinade, preferably overnight.

Get the oil really hot in the wok and then add the garlic and ginger, peeled and finely chopped, and the chilli, also chopped. These seasonings aren't essential, but they do give that authentic Chinese flavour. Now for the vegetables – you can use just two or three, but I like to use quite a lot. Start off with root vegetables and any others that take quite a long time to cook, and work progressively through to the softest ones. First of all put in a finely chopped onion. Stir immediately – the important point is this continual stirring movement. Now add the carrot, very thinly sliced. Always slice vegetables very thinly or cut into matchstick strips because the ingredients have to cook quickly, and they need to be slightly undercooked to preserve a nice texture. I would now add, say, a green pepper and a celery stalk, cut into thin matchstick strips. Just move them all the way round the pan on the highest possible heat. At this stage you can add items like a bit of cauliflower or purple sprouting broccoli. Include the stalks, quite chunkily cut, to give a nice 'bite'. Obviously the heads will take less time to cook, so they'll be much softer. A handful of freshly podded peas would be good here. At this point the stir-fry will start to look very colourful, with a wonderful combination of orange, green, yellow and white. Now add the marinaded chicken pieces. Push the vegetables slightly to one side and tip the chicken into the middle. As soon as it turns opaque add the last ingredients, such as a sliced courgette, some shredded lettuce and a chopped tomato, plus the rest of the marinade and $\frac{1}{4}$ pint (150 ml) of chicken stock made with the stock cube and hot water. Stir for about one minute only, until the sauce is slightly thick and glossy. Serve on a bed of plain boiled rice, or jazz up the rice with a little fried onion or garlic.

VARIATIONS

There is no end to the number of different vegetables and combinations you can use in this basic recipe. Try chicken with broccoli, or chicken with courgettes, or chicken with green peppers. Add a few almonds or walnuts for texture and flavour. It's a good way of using up the end of a cucumber, or the outer leaves of a lettuce which you would normally just throw away because they are too tough for salads. Fish can be substituted for the chicken, but be careful because it needs so little cooking in this very hot pan. Any of the cheaper fishes, such as mackerel, cut into very thin finger strips, are very good. Vegetarians can omit the fish or meat and still have a very tasty, nutritious dish.

SPRING IN NEW YORK

Helene Hanff is the author of 84 Charing Cross Road.* *She
sends monthly reports to* Woman's Hour *from New York, whose famous
Central Park contains a Shakespeare Garden filled with flowers grown from
seedlings sent by listeners*

A hundred thousand New Yorkers ought to send thank you notes
to former Mayor John Lindsay. He changed their lives. Back in
1966, Lindsay was inaugurated on a freezing January day – at the
beginning of a transport strike. For two icy weeks, with no buses
or subways running, people who lived several miles from their
offices couldn't get to work. Lindsay gave the strikers their pay
increase, but he won a concession in return. Thereafter, their
contracts would expire not on 1 January but on 1 April.

Well, in 1980 – on 1 April – the transport workers struck again.
But this time it was spring. The joggers began jogging to work;
other New Yorkers began cycling and roller-skating to work; and
people who had never walked further than the nearest bus-stop
discovered they had feet, and began walking to work. Some of
them went along the major avenues. But for the next two weeks,
early in the morning and late in the afternoon, the 840 acres of
Central Park were sprinkled with joggers, cyclists, skaters and
walkers who were just in time to goggle at the sea of white apple
blossom, followed by the flowering of the white cherry trees. The
strike was over by the time the lilac and the Japanese pink cherry
were in bloom, but the cyclists, skaters and walkers were still in
the park to see them. Since the day the strike ended the number
of riders on New York buses and subways has dropped by 100,000
a day.

The dogs are also out in force, enjoying the spring. You see
them going into the cleaner's, the hardware store, the delicatessen,
but mostly you see them tied by their leashes to the parking meters
at kerbs in front of supermarkets. Some dogs enjoy being tied
there, to watch the passing parade. Some dogs do *not* enjoy it.
Take the dachshund who's been out walking with his mother and
the baby. He notices that while his mother left him and the pram
outside the supermarket, she took the baby in with her. The
dachshund suspects he's been something of a nuisance to her since
the baby came, and he wouldn't put it past her to sneak out of a

back door with the baby and move to Pittsburgh. So he sends up a shrill, angry barking, the gist of which is: 'I know you're in there!' Then there's the Irish setter, owned by a young couple. He has complete faith in their constancy – and no faith at all in their ability to remember where they left him. So he barks, loudly and anxiously, to remind them that they brought him, and to provide them with his exact location. It is the acid test of a writer's love of dogs, to be typing by her open window, with the dachshund and the Irish setter side by side at parking meters directly below the window.

New York breaks out in a rash of block parties in spring and summer. One block will bake things, and make things, to raise money to plant trees on the block. A long avenue will hold a party to call attention to its neighbourhood stores. But I never pass a block party without remembering the spring when our Democratic Club got carried away, and decided to hold its annual fund-raising dinner-dance on a city street – like a block party. There were a few Cassandras who warned that something would go wrong, that we'd forget something essential, but we paid no heed to them.

In true block-party fashion, we got a permit from City Hall to use a side street, lined with old brownstone houses, and a permit from the Police Department to close the street to traffic. We ordered elegant takeaway dinners from a fancy restaurant; and on the great day we set up hired tables along both sidewalks, we put candles and flowers on every table, and set a record-player out in the middle of the street to play music for dancing. At seven o'clock on a May Saturday evening we assembled, two hundred strong, the women in long gowns, and the men, including judges, congressmen and city council men, in full evening dress.

All went swimmingly until coffee was served. It was then that a gentleman rose, sought out a member of the dinner committee, leaned down and asked her a confidential question. At the question, her face froze in horror. When she finally answered, the gentleman's face froze in complete panic. The word the gentleman used was 'john', but I'll translate it. The question he asked was 'Where's the loo?' The answer he got was: 'There isn't any.' For the rest of the long, long evening, dignified judges and learned counsels, in their formal evening clothes, could be seen haggling with the janitors of brownstone rooming-houses, to whom they paid steadily rising prices for the use of ancient, insanitary loos in tenement basements. If the gentlemen had been in any condition to walk three long cross-town blocks, I could have made a fortune renting out my bathroom.

*Published by Deutsch/Futura

DO'S AND DON'TS OF DRESSMAKING

Betty Foster runs a design studio in Crewe and has had a TV series on dressmaking. Here she explains the right order in which to tackle dressmaking, and includes some expert tips as well as instructions for fitting a basic pattern

If walking through a good fabric department doesn't inspire you to sew, I don't think anything could. However a lot of people aren't sure how to put patterns and fabrics together, and don't know whether to buy the pattern and then the fabric, or vice versa. A beginner should look at ready-made clothes to see how manufacturers relate their styles to the most suitable materials. A draped garment, for instance, will be made up in a soft, fluid material, and never in a crisp fabric more appropriate for tailored styles. There are basically two different types of fabrics: first, the familiar woven ones which sew beautifully, press well, and are often used for fitted garments; and second, the great range of knitted fabrics, all of which stretch, and therefore drape very well. Some of them can, however, be very difficult to handle, especially the fine, slippery polyesters and cotton jerseys, which can create problems on the sewing machine. You need a machine that will do a very small, scarcely visible zig-zag stitch, or one with a special stitch for sewing stretch fabrics.

Just as important as the right stitch is the right thread. Take your fabric to the haberdashery department and ask their advice. Look at the fabric before you buy it to see whether it has to be cut in a single direction – it may affect how much you buy. If you have sewn before, you may have found that you have fabric left over. Work out why – are you short, perhaps? You may be able to buy less than the pattern states, and save the price of your zip and other bits and pieces.

If the fabric is liable to seat or can be seen through, you should line it. Buy a lining material that relates in quality to the price of the main fabric, because if it wears out long before the garment it's a waste of money. The cuffs and collar, and the front edges where the buttons and buttonholes are going, may need an inter-facing too. It goes between the lining and the main fabric, and must be the right weight. Ask advice at the time. Don't leave your material folded, but buy a fabric roller or make one from news-paper or brown paper; it will make for easier cutting out in due course.

Before you start to sew, take out your sewing machine and make sure it's thoroughly cleaned: remove all the fluff from around the spool case and anywhere else; if you have to oil the machine, follow the instructions in the manual very carefully. If it's an electric machine, check the wires in the plug. Make sure the machine is functioning properly by practising on old scraps of material all the things you do when making a garment. I have two small pieces of fabric joined to leave enough of an opening for a very short zip – it can be one from an old garment – which I regularly put in to make sure that I won't be struggling with the real thing.

Modern, man-made fabrics give machine needles quite a ham-mering and you need to change them more often than with natural fabrics. Ideally you should have a new one for each garment. Make sure before you start that you have the right needle for the job – you will need ballpoint needles, for example, for difficult knitted and stretch fabrics, and for suede and leather special needles with a spade blade that goes through easily.

If you think your machine is inadequate and want a new one, compare all the different models in the shops, and make sure that you're going to get all the operations you need – at the very least good forward and reverse, easy change to swing needle, and the ability to do buttonholes easily, quickly and proficiently. Buy from a reliable source, so that you can go back for help and advice if necessary.

Now for other tools of the trade. Throw away any rusty pins, because they can mark and badly damage fabric. If you're buying new pins, have stainless steel ones. I find the longer pins easy to pick up and handle; a lot of people like the pins with coloured knobs on the end, which you can see easily in the fabric and on the carpet. A magnetic pin box is a good idea. Good scissors can be very expensive, but are a marvellous investment. They have to be sharp, they must cut easily, and they should feel right in your hand. Modern fabrics blunt them very easily, so find out if they can be resharpened; if yours have gone blunt, get them sharpened before you start dressmaking.

Once you've decided what you're going to make, you need a paper pattern, which must correspond to your shape, size and ability. Before you look at pattern books take your bust, waist and hip measurements, and check your height in stockinged feet. Pattern books include seven size charts, which cover different heights as well as measurements round the body; one of the categories may fit you better than the others. Buy a dress pattern by your bust measurement, and skirt and trouser patterns by your hip measurement, because you can alter the waist more easily.

If you are nowhere near a standard size, and such people are in the majority, have yourself measured properly by somebody else, because you need a few extra measurements. Then buy a basic pattern, which is a dress that's all in one at the front, with darts for the waist and bust, two pieces for the back, and inset sleeves. Use your own measurements to adjust the pattern as near as possible to yourself. Try it out first in some cheap fabric or a remnant. I often try out basic patterns in non-woven interfacing fabric, because it's cheap. I can pin it together and try it against myself, but I haven't wasted the material because I can use it for interfacing collars and so on.

With a correct basic pattern you have two alternatives. You can use it to alter other patterns by putting your personal pattern down with the new one on top, and bringing them into line; but more important, a good basic pattern enables you to learn how to make other styles from it, which is much simpler than you think. If you want to learn more about this, try your local evening classes. The important thing to remember is that the pattern must be right before the scissors go in, because that's the point of no return.

Now you are ready to cut out. You may want to cut out on your own, but I prefer having somebody with me to watch what I'm doing, help me fold the material, and perhaps work from the other side of the table. You can use the floor to cut out on, but I do it on a table, though not on the actual table top. I went to a do-it-yourself shop and had a 3×4 ft (90×115 cm) piece of hard-board cut; I then covered the rough side with a very cheap felt. If I put the board felt side down on my dining-table it does no damage, and I've got an excellent smooth cutting surface; if I've got slippery material, however, I put the smooth surface straight down on to the kitchen table and cut out on the felt side, so that the material doesn't slide about.

Hold the fabric up with one end to the ground and the other end upwards into the air, so that you can see if there's the slightest change of colour, or if the flowers go all one way, or if it has to be cut in one direction only. Look for faults, because a small flaw could ruin the look of the garment. If you spot it beforehand you can possibly avoid it in the cutting out or put it in an inconspicuous place.

Fold the fabric, following the cutting instructions on the pattern. At one end of my table I usually put a chair, on which I place the fabric, which I then pull, folded, into position on the table. First of all I lay on to it all the large pattern pieces, watching the grain lines very carefully, and pinning the pieces very firmly into place, at right-angles to the cutting edge, which I keep well away from. I usually have a second chair at the other end to receive the fabric, and then when I've finished all the pinning I can bring the fabric slowly back up on to the table and start cutting out.

I keep the leftover bits and use tailor's chalk to mark an arrow indicating the cutting direction. Then if I need to cut a piece again, or want an extra bit of fabric, I don't have to work out which way I was cutting originally. I leave the pattern on the fabric until it's all cut out and I've transferred all the necessary pattern markings. Are the notches there, to make me match the seams correctly? Have I marked all the darts? Have I marked the button and buttonhole positions? I use tailor's chalk pencils, not the flat, blunt kind, because the pencils come in different colours and you can also sharpen them, which makes them more economical and gives more positive marking.

Finally I take some leftovers and try the fabric on my machine. I make sure I've got the stitch length right. I decide whether I need to use a slightly zig-zag stitch – knitted fabrics, for instance, will need one. I also see what heat I've got to set the iron at to press the fabric well. The actual sewing is quick and easy if you have cut out properly.

WHAT THE BUDGET MEANS

What does the Budget mean to the average tax-payer and consumer?
Journalist Frances Cairncross explains what lies behind some of the
statements the Chancellor of the Exchequer makes in his annual Budget speech

The Budget is a peculiar part of the British financial ritual which doesn't take place in other countries in quite the same way. What's very odd about it from my point of view is the fact that it is basically about tax. In the past, the Government has planned its public spending usually for as much as five years ahead, though it rarely sticks to those plans. Then it comes to the country with great fanfares and says, 'This is how we're going to pay for it.' But the public spending part of the exercise has all gone on before – it's rather as if you or I went off and decided what we were going to spend for the next five years on clothes, houses, cars, food or whatever, and then said how we were going to earn enough to pay for it all. This very topsy-turvy way of doing things doesn't happen in other countries, who usually plan their public spending and tax changes at the same time.

One of the things which affects taxation in Britain very much indeed is what is happening to inflation, though it has different effects on income tax from those it has on the duties with which we are all familiar – those on tobacco and alcohol. Tobacco and alcohol are in a way the easiest effects to understand. If the duty on a bottle of whisky is, say, about £3 a bottle, as inflation drives up the price of the whisky itself it means that the duty, in relation to the price of the final bottle of whisky, becomes a smaller proportion of the total. If the Chancellor does nothing at all, the amount of money he collects in duty is worth less because inflation has whittled it away. So every year the Chancellor really has to raise the duty on whisky and tobacco simply to take account of the way in which inflation is reducing the purchasing power of the duty on these commodities. Why the Government hasn't arranged for an automatic adjustment of these duties so that they always keep step with inflation, I don't know.

The effect that inflation has on the income tax we pay is slightly harder to understand, but roughly speaking what happens is this. If it is left as it is, the value of the income tax allowance you get each year is eroded by inflation. Although the allowance you get may stay at £1,000 – just to pluck a figure out of the air – from one year to the next, you are actually paying more tax because the value of that allowance has been eroded by rising prices. A few years ago an amendment was tacked on to a finance bill, stating that the Chancellor *must* raise tax allowances in line with rising prices in the past year, unless during his Budget speech he specifically said he was not going to do so. That had a very salutary effect on Chancellors. Until then, they had tended to declare that they were generously going to raise personal tax allowances; everyone then thought they were going to pay less tax, but in fact they paid exactly the same amount of tax relative to their total income. What was happening was that they were finding their tax bill increased by the surreptitious effect of inflation. Now, if they want to raise income tax, they must come clean about it.

CHEESE SOUFFLÉ

Mary Berry's recipe serves three people

1½ oz (40 g) butter
1½ oz (40 g) flour
½ pint (300 ml) milk
salt
pepper
7 level teaspoons made mustard
4 oz (125 g) strong Cheddar cheese, or 3 oz (90 g) Cheddar and
    1 oz (30 g) Parmesan
4 large eggs
pinch of nutmeg

Pre-heat the oven to 375°F (190°C, gas mark 5), and place a baking sheet in it. Melt the butter in a pan, stir in the flour, and cook for 2 minutes, without browning, to make a roux. Heat the milk in another pan. Remove the roux pan from the heat and stir in the hot milk. Return to the heat and bring to the boil. Stir until thickened, then add the seasoning and mustard and leave to cool. Grate the cheese and stir in. Separate the eggs and beat the yolks one at a time into the cheese sauce. Whisk the whites with a rotary hand or electric whisk until stiff but not dry. Stir 1 heaped tablespoon into the cheese sauce and then carefully fold in the remainder. Pour into a buttered, 2 pint (1.25 l) soufflé dish, run a teaspoon around the edge, and bake on the hot baking sheet in the centre of the oven for about 40 minutes, until well risen and golden brown.

VARIATIONS

Choose any flavouring and add to the mixture before the egg yolks.

Ham: Add 4 to 6 oz (125 to 175 g) ham or boiled bacon, finely chopped.

Fish: Add 4 to 6 oz (125 to 175 g) finely flaked, cooked smoked haddock.

Shellfish: Add 4 oz (125 g) peeled prawns or shrimps.

Mushrooms: Add 8 oz (250 g) finely chopped mushrooms sautéd in 1 oz (30 g) butter.

Spinach: Add 1 lb (500 g) cooked, finely chopped spinach with a pinch of nutmeg, topped with a little grated cheese.

GROWING YOUR OWN COURGETTES AND SWEETCORN

Television gardening expert Clay Jones explains how best to cultivate these delicious summer vegetables

You can sow courgette seed in a greenhouse, or in a propagator in the kitchen – somewhere warm. Alternatively when the danger of frosts is over, about the beginning of June, you can plant seed outside in fertile soil.

I have developed a method for getting more courgettes per plant which involves, about mid-April, digging out a hole 2 feet square, and 18 inches to 2 feet deep. In the bottom of the hole put as much fresh manure or garden compost as you can, and you can mix in with it some fresh lawn clippings, providing of course that the lawn hasn't been recently treated with a weedkiller. What you're creating is a hot bed. Put a foot of that beautiful stuff at the bottom, then replace the soil on top until it's level with the surrounding surface again. But don't press it down. If it sinks more than 3 inches put some more soil back on top, so that finally you've got a bowl 3 inches in depth.

Round about the second or third week in May put in the middle of that bowl two courgette seeds. Sow them about ½ inch apart on end or on edge, and hide them about ½ inch. Then get a 1 lb or 2 lb jam jar and place it upside-down over them to make a tiny greenhouse. Any sun is of course trapped by the jar, and it really heats up the soil. Germination takes place within about seven to ten days. If both seeds have germinated remove the weaker of the two and leave the other one to grow on. Take away the jam jar, otherwise it will strangle the growth of the courgette plant.

During the growing season, unless it's pouring with rain and the soil is absolutely saturated, really soak that trough the moment the surface appears dry – 2 gallons of water is not too much, and 4 gallons at a time will probably be right. Because the courgette is a very large-leaved plant, the fruit needs a lot of water in order to form.

If you suspect that disease is going to be a problem, prevent it by spraying beforehand, and this is something that applies to all vegetables. Also, if in a certain year any vegetable has suffered from some kind of pest or disease, the following year move it as far away as you can. This is the whole basis of crop rotation – because of the danger of a build-up of diseases and pests, move the plant. There are two varieties of courgette which I find are worth growing – Zucchini and Golden Zucchini.

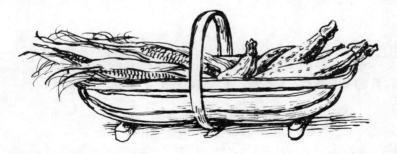

Sweetcorn is becoming a popular vegetable to grow in the garden, and like everything else it needs plenty of food and water to produce big plants. But with sweetcorn there's also a special secret. Imagine the sweetcorn plant – a six-foot-tall, stately, upright plant that doesn't branch very much. The male flowers are borne right on top and down beneath are the female flowers. Sweetcorn belongs to the same family as grasses, and the pollen is very light indeed. Therefore if you plant your sweetcorn in one straight row, any breeze from any direction will carry the pollen away from the female flowers underneath, and you're not going to get any crops. The way to get over that is to plant them in rectangular blocks, so that no matter which way the breeze is coming from, some pollen will always hit the female flowers.

You can grow the plants outside in the same way as for courgettes. But because I want my plants to come into flower as early as possible, so that the late summer sun will ripen the crop, I like to start them early under glass or in a propagator at about 55° to 60°F. An important thing to remember about sweetcorn is that it absolutely hates being transplanted. I get fibre pots, put in them some soilless compost, sow one seed per pot smack in the middle, keep the pots moist at the temperature mentioned, and just let them grow in that. If you can't plant them out when they should be planted out, feed them in the pots to keep them going, but eventually round about the end of May or the beginning of June, when the frosts have gone, plant out the whole thing. The root will come through the bottom of the pot into the soil and the plant won't even know you've moved it.

As for diseases, sweetcorn is as tough as old boots and hardly ever has any problems. Early King is obviously an early variety, and there's an old one which I still grow called Kelvedon Wonder. Aztec is a new one which I have tried recently and I was quite pleased with it.

GROWING VEGETABLES FOR SHOW

Bill Taylor has held the United Kingdom onion record and is familiar with the highly competitive world of growing super-veg and with dastardly tricks like nocturnal leek-slashing. Geoff Amos is technical editor of Garden News

The old-fashioned leek grower's time-honoured ritual on show day began some time between half past five and seven o'clock, when he dug up his leeks and picked the two best ones for exhibiting later that day. Then every leaf would be washed and cleaned, and the outside of the leeks wiped with a cloth dipped in the top of the milk to give them a rich sheen. Breakfast had to be a movable feast, for the kitchen was totally given over to the leeks.

Bill Taylor talked about the thrill he felt on the morning of a show. 'It's an inborn excitement, because over the summer and the previous winter you've been working up to this high point. Suddenly there you are with your specimens, going up to the tent. It really grips you. If you look at the other exhibitors they're all hypnotized by it, too. It's a marvellous experience. You take a furtive glance round to see what the others have got, and you do all sorts of little things to make your exhibit look nice; it's officially called presentation, but I say it's catching the judge's eye.' To demonstrate his point Bill produced an onion 19 inches in circumference and weighing $4\frac{3}{4}$ lb. It was dry all round, of a uniform colour, and fully ripened. Such an eye-catching onion is produced by pulling off the broken skins while it is growing; the sun and nature do the rest.

Geoff Amos explained what the judge hopes to find. 'He doesn't look for great size at the expense of quality, so he won't fall over backwards when he sees the biggest onion there. If it's a class for six onions, he has to look for uniformity, and for nice skins, as Bill said, with no cracks in them. He feels the tops to see if they're soft – if they are, they may be bad inside, but he doesn't cut them open. He can tell from experience if the onion is good all the way through. I would pick it up and hold it in my hand – I could tell by the weight. I would also press round the top of the stem to see if it was soft.'

Bill produced a gigantic leek some three feet long. In spite of what some people think, these enormous vegetables are not grown at the expense of taste. He told us how to cultivate good leeks from your own seed. 'If you sow a packet of leek seeds you might have one or two that are bigger than the rest. Eat all the others, but let the big ones stay in the ground over the winter, so that they come up next July into a flower head. Each little flower will be pollinated by bees, and then start to make seeds. What I do to get a large, early leek is this. At the beginning of July, when these heads are all coming out into flower, I take a pair of nail scissors and clip off the bottom two layers of little flowers. The plant will be fertilized by bees on the top, but it has to do something about this little space at the bottom, so it forms bulbils, which are little green shoots two or three inches long. At the base of each of these will be a minature onion. About the end of October take these shoots into your greenhouse, and put each one into an old milk bottle containing some water. Round about Christmas they will have thickened out and you can just pull them off. At the bottom of each you will see a tiny bulb which you plant in peat compost for cuttings, in an ordinary seed tray, about an inch apart; they will then root. They don't need much heat – no more than 45° to 50°F. Leave them there until they start growing, then transplant them into a larger box, put that into a tall frame, and plant them out at the end of April.'

The giant show leeks weren't grown underground, Bill went on to explain, like the normal ones. He plants them at ground level and then puts lantiles – land drains – over the leek so that a third of the leaf is over the top. They get fed and watered in the usual way, but are growing in a tube above ground to make them really big and keep them clean.

Geoff mentioned some other vegetables that are grown for showing. 'Celery, although it's a bog plant and likes plenty of rain, can have too much rain, which causes it to go rotten in the centre.' Peas and beans are favourites for showing, of course, but a class for the longest bean doesn't leave much room for the judge's discretion. More interesting to Geoff, because they help to develop vegetable gardening, are classes for a dozen peas on a plate, for instance, or half a dozen runner beans, or a plate of beetroot. It's helpful to know what sort of judge you're dealing with – if it is the greengrocer at the end of the street, the largest will do; but if he's from the Royal Horticultural Society or the National Vegetable Society, it's a different kettle of fish. The Royal Horticultural Society judges are very experienced gardeners, and though Bill Taylor hasn't always agreed with some of their decisions against him, he's always given in to them because he regards them as the ultimate in judges.

We hear a lot about vandalism and cheating taking place before big competitions, and Bill confirmed that it did indeed happen. 'People come round and steal your stuff, or mark it, or get a knife and cut it. Some people are so jealous, which I can't understand because gardening is a friendly occupation. I've had it done to me

36

repeatedly – they've cut away my onions, pushed them, put their feet on them and trodden them down. They've pulled my runner beans out of the rows so that they've been spoilt. I could go on for a long while. . . .' On this subject Geoff made another point, which is that showmen save the seed from their onions. If a rival sees that your onions are bigger than his, he may come along at dead of night and steal those onions so that he can grow that strain from seed himself. Bill agreed that this had happened to him in the past.

The great value of horticultural shows is that they help both the competitors and the amateur gardeners. Standards were rising constantly, Geoff said, and strains were being improved; and people in general were showing a greater interest in gardening, something that always happens at a time of economic decline.

DRINKS ON THE LAWN

Has Anne Jones got the only teetotal slugs in Britain?

Let me give every gardener a piece of advice – though I wouldn't dream of being so bossy were it not for the fact that we are continually being told by experts to do this thing. And it is quite wrong. What I am most strongly advising is this: DO NOT SERVE BEER TO YOUR SLUG.

Slugs plural, really. They don't come in ones. They come in herds, droves, like stampeding beeves in cowboy films – or locusts, devouring everything that gets in their way. That's slugs – a cross between a locust and a beef. And what we are always being advised to do is give them beer. Every gardening magazine and every gardening programme advocates beer in saucers, as slug traps. Slug pellets are rather frowned on, the theory being that the slugs eat them and then die a horrible death. It's no fun being a slug, I can see that. Anyway, apparently when they have breathed their last birds come along and eat them, and then they die, too. Worse than that is the danger that children might pick up the pellets from the soil and eat them before the slugs get a chance. This theory has been disproved recently, though, by the manufacturers, whose research reveals that children hardly ever pick them up off the soil but eat them straight from the packet.

So, like me, you may incline to the beer trap idea. Small saucers of beer, say the experts, placed strategically around the garden, are irresistible to slugs. They come for miles at the first whiff of the hop, drink the beer, get drunk, fall in and die a happy death – it is assumed. Anyway, I opened a can of beer, filled a saucer, and placed it, strategically, in the garden. (It was light ale, by the way; I don't know if this is significant, and I mention it only for scientific purposes.) There it sat, like a pool of liquid sunshine. Two days later, there it still sat. Total absence of slugs – alive, dead or drunk.

Perhaps I was a bit impatient. I suppose just one saucer of beer wasn't likely to over-excite the entire slug population of east Surrey. At the same time I did have a certain curiosity to witness a slug actually quaffing beer from a saucer. So I went and found a slug and transported it by hand to the beer. It took a single sniff, screwed up its little face, and backed off. Thinking it didn't quite understand the situation, I put it back. Same thing again, only faster – well, by slug standards. I put it back yet again; in fact I put its nose right into the beer – and I could swear it quivered with distaste. I could almost hear it saying primly: 'Not for me, thank you. I'll just have a tomato juice.' (I bet it would have, too: and the tomato – indeed the entire tomato plant, given half a chance.) 'Just one sip, to please me', I said. It took no notice. 'You're a fool to yourself, slug', I said. 'Listen. You like beer. All the gardening people say so. Now drink up!'

Finally I picked up the slug and put it right into the beer. Total immersion. I am not proud of this. Here I was, deliberately trying to drown a slug in cold blood – or rather cold beer. So, I went away and gave it five minutes to guzzle itself comatose. . . . After which I found that the slug had swum out of the beer, out of the saucer, and was cantering away at a rate of knots. . . . I let it go – I know when I'm beaten.

But what can be the meaning of this? I cannot believe that I have the only swimming, teetotal slug in the world in my garden. Can it be, then, that all slugs are in fact amphibious non-drinkers, and the saucer-of-beer theory only a cunning story put about by the breweries, to boost sales? On the other hand, could it be that I happened to tangle with a specially pernickety slug, who preferred milk stout, say? Or a very well-mannered slug, who didn't care to drink from the saucer? But I can't be pandering to the whims of a slug, can I? What did it expect? A beer mat? Crisps?

TRAVELS OF A PLANT HUNTER IN KASHMIR

*Tree specialist Roy Lancaster describes an expedition to the foothills of the Himalayas**

We flew into Srinagar, the capital of Kashmir, and spent the first two days on Lake Dal, which is the usual beginning to a Kashmir holiday. The lake has some lovely houseboats on it, surrounded by rafts of beautiful water-lilies and lotus flowers. The lotus is like a many-petalled pink tulip, with a long stem which rises gracefully out of the water; imagine a giant-sized nasturtium leaf coming out of the water, and that's the lotus leaf. And jewelled kingfishers kept spinning past. It's like something out of paradise.

We were shown floating islands – allotments, really. Vegetation was raked up from the bottom of the lake and stabilized with great props so that vegetables could be planted on it; we were told that rustlers came in the night by boat, hooked on to the end of an island, cut the ropes which held it, and then paddled away with the vegetable garden! Can you imagine somebody paddling away with your vegetable patch in Britain?

I shall never forget the morning we emerged from our hotel to go on our first trip into the forest on ponies. Outside was a great crowd of ponies and pony-boys, making a tremendous din. Then one of our number, a very forthright lady of the British Empire type, said, 'I know about ponies. I'll go and sort them out and make sure we don't have any duffs.' So she strode forward, but that was also the signal for all the pony-boys to surge forward, too. Several people fell to the ground, and one rather large lady ended up astride two ponies. After about a quarter of an hour seated on my pony I looked around and counted the party – thankfully, they were all there. Off we set in a cloud of dust like the sheriff's posse in a Western.

We rode along through the woods amid the sweet smell of pines, firs and spruces – giant specimens, all of them. Eventually, as we

39

climbed, we left the woods behind and reached the alpine mead-ows. There in a snow gully we saw beautiful, white, six-foot-high foxtail lilies and all manner of alpine plants. But the main problem at that stage was that goats and other grazing animals had beaten us to it; that was always the difficulty in Kashmir – to get there before the grazing animals which eat everything down to ground level. It wasn't until later in the tour that we were to see the Kashmir alpines at their very best.

There are several Mogul gardens there – gardens planted by the Mogul emperors four hundred years ago. I suppose the Shalimar is the most famous, and a number of us had jokingly thought we would stand outside the walls and sing that old-time song about them that goes, 'Pale hands I loved. . . .' But when we got there it was a very different story. The Shalimar Gardens were derelict, the beds were weedy, the fountains weren't working, and the lakes and canals in which the fountains were situated were full of drying mud. One of the famous trees had been blown down in a very powerful gale the previous night. In the village of Shalimar we found a huge specimen of the chennar tree – the oriental plane, which is a parent of the London plane found in the streets of many British cities. This was an absolute giant, with a lower trunk rather like an elephant's foot. It was the focal point of the village, where all the meetings were held and local gossip was exchanged.

We passed through there on our way to Sonnamag, which was really wonderful. The white Kashmir birch stood out like a ghost in the mists at early morning and late in the evening. It's much whiter than the silver birch we know in Europe – in fact it looks as if it's been whitewashed. I brought some of the seed back and I now have a tiny Kashmir birch tree in my lawn, planted in 1978.

We also went by pony into the mountains to a place called Vishensa, where there was a lake into which some forgotten son of the Raj had at some stage put brown trout – so we had trout for breakfast. There the alpine flowers flowed right into the camp, came into the tents and tickled our toes. We had two rapturous days in that perfect paradise of flowers which carpeted the ground at our feet – anemones, gentians, primulas of many kinds and dwarf rhododendrons, in all the colours you could possibly imagine and in great profusion.

*His book *Plant Hunting in Nepal* is published by Croom Helm

CLICHÉS OF STAGE, SCREEN AND RADIO

Anne Garvey

For some playwrights and screenwriters, answering the door or telephone emerges as a major drama. 'Who can that be at this time of night?' cry the actors wondrously. The fact that it's meant to be only 8.30 never deters them. And then there's the time-honoured opening of: 'Oh, it's you. You'd better come in', which is exclusively a TV/radio phrase, unknown to the outside world, who in my observation take knocks at the door in their stride.

Some of the clichés are blatant padding popped in to plump out the plot, like the 'I didn't hear you properly' ploy. The writer's running short on dialogue, so he slips in this 'Tell me again' technique to fill things out a bit. You know the sort of thing. Diana tells her husband she has a lover. She explains it clearly enough in her ringing RADA voice and we're all agog to know how the husband will react. Will he leave her, knock her down, laugh uproariously or what? He does none of these things. Instead he says, 'I don't understand what you're saying, Diana', or 'What does all this mean? Who is this man you're talking about?'; or, more simply, he pours himself one of those huge drinks they're always downing on TV plays, then says, 'Tell me what's wrong, Diana.' So we get Diana's saga all over again when a child of four could have got the gist of it in the first place. I swear this kind of thing has kept *The Archers* going for so long. No one ever gets the message, and it all takes so long. 'Hang on a minute now, young Neil. Hold your horses. You're telling me that the pig unit is on fire?'

Do the producers really think we poor dim listeners can't follow what's going on, or is it that they're too lazy not to pull these tired old clichés out of the bag every time there's a lull? No one ever listens to anyone in radio and TV dramas. No wonder. If you've got ten minutes' worth of dialogue that you need to spin out to twenty, it helps if no one communicates with anyone else. In fact, it's very convenient. 'Oh, I say, there's Margot running along the cliff top. She looks upset.' Indeed she is. Death lurks only yards from the heroes' feet, yet Margot's inarticulacy is the heart of the play. She blusters, fumes, and points wildly to the cliff edge. Our heroes interrogate Margot: 'What can be the matter?' But she still can't manage it and off they stride amid mounting background music towards that fatal spot.

Why can't she simply say there's a fifty-foot drop over the next hill, or the vicar is waiting for you with a loaded gun? In real life anyone, however distraught, would manage to spit it out, but not the Margots of television plays. At times of great agitation when someone – usually a woman – has something really vital to say, they never get a chance to speak out sensibly. Instead they're told, with astonishing regularity, to try and get some rest. Rest is manifestly the last thing they want or need, but the instruction pops up invariably at times of crisis. 'You're overwrought', the actors beam cheerfully. 'Try and get some rest.' Or marginally more infuriating: 'You can tell us all about it later. First Peter and I must go to the village and talk to the vicar. Seems a friendly enough sort of bloke.' Now we know, and so does poor inarticulate Margot, that the vicar is far from friendly and that he's waiting behind the drawing-room door with his Colt .45. But if communications were better and Margot did manage to choke out her awful warning, where would the rest of the plot be? If the investigators actually listened and didn't keep their appointment with the gun-toting clergyman, what would happen to the paper-thing storyline?

Procrastination is the stock-in-trade of so much drama, and television characters are quite unlike real-life people. 'Let's talk about it in the morning', our hero calls airily. Doesn't he know there's not going to be any morning for him, unless he hears her out now and finds out that the escaped werewolf is only half a mile from the house? Hasn't he seen any of these plays? He can't have, or he couldn't suggest that most infuriating strategy of the lot: 'I'll take a look around. You stay here and let no one in, do you hear?' We know it won't work. The predictability of the scene to come doesn't make it any less frightening, though. In fact, it irritatingly increases the fear stakes. I can't bear the 'Let's separate' routine and always switch off; I just don't think I can stand going through it all over again. We all know that the werewolf is by this time actually in the basement, and what with her friend going off to take a look around – taking the gun with him, of course – there's little hope for the heroine. It's all rather wearing, but we put up with it.

We tolerate many more clichés, many more fictions and departures from true human response than the programme-makers give us credit for. In fact we're quite kind to them on the whole, but they shouldn't think that we don't know what they're doing, or that we haven't noticed, because we certainly have. But then, to quote one of my favourite clichés: 'I just don't know. I don't know anything any more.'

WHEATMEAL BREAD

Mary Berry's recipe makes a 2 lb loaf and four rolls, and only needs one rising

Yeast mixture
¾ pint (400 ml) hand-hot water
1 level teaspoon sugar
1 level tablespoon dried yeast

Dough
12 oz (350 g) strong plain flour
12 oz (350 g) wholemeal flour
2 to 3 teaspoons salt
1 tablespoon salad oil

To make the yeast mixture mix the water and sugar and stir in the dried yeast. Leave to stand for 10 to 15 minutes until frothy.

To make the dough put all the remaining ingredients in a bowl. Pour on the yeast mixture and oil and mix with a fork, then knead until smooth and no longer sticky, which will take about 10 minutes. Grease a 2 lb (1 kg) loaf tin. Weigh out 2 lb of the bread dough and divide into four sausage shapes the width of the tin. Lay them in the tin and put the whole lot in a large polythene bag. Shape the remaining dough into four bread rolls, place on a well-greased baking sheet and put that in another polythene bag.

Leave the bread to rise in a warm kitchen for about an hour or in a cold kitchen for 2 hours. Then the rolls will have doubled in bulk and the bread will have risen to the top of the tin. Pre-heat the oven to 450°F (230°C, gas mark 8). Bake the loaf for about 40 minutes, when it should be evenly browned and sound hollow when tapped on the bottom. The bread rolls will take about 20 minutes.

PERSONAL WONDERS

Every schoolchild used to know the Seven Wonders of the Ancient World. Here four people in the public eye reveal their personal wonders in the modern world. First, writer and critic Andrew Sinclair, who believes that the way we travel is an important factor in understanding our destination

If you want to wonder at a great sight, absorb it, feel part of its time and its history – you must approach it properly, with reverence. Getting there is half of being there. I have had some marvellous experiences, when I've gone on a pilgrimage to a place and become part of what I have seen. Four places really stay with me: the Five Sisters windows of York Minster, Stonehenge, the temple of Machu Picchu in the Andes, and Sigiriya, the Lion Rock of Sri Lanka.

When I went to York I walked for a week from Edinburgh. I slept out, had very little money, and became almost like an animal. I remember particularly sleeping out on Hadrian's Wall and feeling like a Roman sentry, hearing the curlews in the evening and the owls at night, being very cold, and very afraid of the Picts and Scots to the north . . . I was going back through time. By the time I reached York Minster I was almost in a state of hallucination through fatigue and hunger. I looked at the grey windows called the Five Sisters, wondering why they hadn't been smashed like everything else in Cromwell's times. Those beautiful grey glass windows have no image of God, nothing – they are like nothing else in England. A crusader had apparently given them. Why had he given these *grisaille* windows, showing all these shades in the sunset? And suddenly I realized why they were there. Of course – he had seen Islam, and in Islam you cannot show God. There was a man all those years ago, in the thirteenth century, who saw that there might be many ways to God. And this was his particular way of showing it, in a Christian church, at a time when he should have been burnt for doing it.

I remember walking on the sacred way from Glastonbury to

Canterbury, and I timed to pass Stonehenge exactly at the point of the summer solstice. You mustn't go to Stonehenge by car, arriving where two roads fork in front of it, looking across barbed wire. You must walk in four miles from the south, or forty miles from Glastonbury. In the evening you will see the hares going over the cornfields, and terrible chimneys from Larkhill Camp – they have an artillery range among the tombs beyond. Then, as you

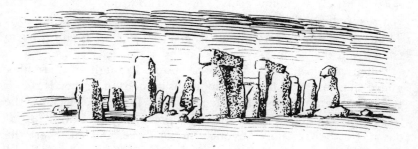

come over the rise, you will see great stone shapes marching from the north. Stone men. On that particular night I saw these stone men marching towards me. They were too far away to see what surrounds them – the barbed wire. I spent a night in the spinney above and came in at dawn. I talked to a very cunning druid in the tea bar afterwards, and thought how artful it was to preserve anything of the past in the present. But the stones themselves, seen from a long way away – those are what mattered, and those are what were alive and had lasted.

The third experience was going to the temple of Machu Picchu. You take a little railway all the way across the top of the Andes, but don't go back on it, as they say. I stayed overnight at the little hotel, and then got up at dawn, before anyone else, and went out to the sacrifice stone. I was very lucky that morning, because a blood-red sun came up across the Andes, and I could see the point of the heart-shaped sacrifice stone, pointing straight at that sun. Suddenly, as I looked around, I could see that every single stone was set in an alignment with the hills and everything else. I knew that I was in one of the great observatories. Again I felt all alone there, and that I was part of a great chain of the living and the dead. And I felt how human blood, in a way, binds us through time.

The last of the places which have given me strange journeys

through time and made me feel part of them was in Sri Lanka, or Ceylon, as it used to be called. I went to the great Lion Rock of Sigiriya, which sticks up about three thousand feet from the middle of a plain. A king of Ceylon was once walled up and starved to death by his younger son. The elder son fled away to southern India. The younger son built this fortress because, since he was guilty of parricide, he was afraid of his brother coming from the north with an avenging army. He filled the Lion Rock with ten years' supplies of food and water. He was absolutely impregnable. Then he sat there for eighteen years, waiting for his brother to come from the north.

When you go up the Lion Rock you go through an incredible guard chamber with beautiful maidens planted in it, then through two 'Ozymandias' legs fifty feet high – just legs, because the statue has collapsed, as in Shelley's poem. Again I went up at dawn, two hours before anyone else got there, and sat where the king had sat for eighteen years and looked towards India. I looked across a pleasure garden he had laid out in the shape of a dead man, with pools for eyes. It pointed towards India: it was his father's corpse.

Now a strange thing happened. When his brother came with an inferior army from India, this king did not stay in the Lion Rock. He rode out with his vermilion elephants and went to assault his brother. Why? If he had ignored them, his brother's army would have fallen apart. The king had spent all this time setting that situation up, and this was the problem I had to solve. I just sat there a couple of hours until the first people came, and I thought I had the answer. He had sat there all those years, looking towards India, and when his elder brother came it was such a relief. Now the story gets stranger. The younger brother won the battle, but at the point of winning it he turned back his elephant. His army fled, and he was cut to pieces. And I suddenly realized that, after all those years of guilt and waiting, he had gone out to lose gladly. It's an important principle to learn, how to lose gladly as well as want to win.

Do not rush at anything which is great or old or has a message. If you go there slowly – and it will still be very fast compared with how these things were made – you may see something that will change your life.

My very first wonder of the world was a big, soft, half-Angora rabbit called Gillian. I loved this rabbit much more deeply than I loved my baby sister, and for numerous reasons. The rabbit never opened her throat and bawled and took all the attention away from me. The rabbit never got taken up in the middle of the night to be petted and soothed. No, the rabbit just sat there in the hutch patiently and waited for me to come and give her more lettuce and more dandelions each day. The rabbit would snuffle and look up at me with big, adoring, pink eyes, but my sister would screw up her little eyes and bellow if I poked affectionately. And anyway, to have a rabbit was to be something special. Nobody else at school had a rabbit, but baby sisters were two a penny and everyone had them. I used to pray for Gillian's soul and I became very thundery when it was suggested that rabbits might not have souls in the same way that we did. I strongly advised my mother against the new sister that she was preparing me for, and I suggested that we should have a rabbit instead. Another rabbit. All those nice, round, shapeless, fuzzy animals still remain as a wonder to me. I like mad, fuzzy Chinchilla cats, and dogs that are covered in shaggy coats, and small birds before their feathers get sleek. I don't like elegant, understated things – I like a lot of fluff and fuzz.

I think the second wonder for me was seeing the Mediterranean Sea. As a schoolgirl I'd been reading about it for years and years, and everything seemed to have happened in it or on it or at its shores. But nothing prepared me for it and its incredible blueness. It wasn't a bit like the ice-cold Irish Sea which would freeze the legs off you. My school was on a cliff near Dublin, and it was considered very lacking in school spirit and moral fibre, not to mention downright disobedient, if we didn't plunge joyously into the sea for a swim every afternoon of the summer term. We were always being told that every other schoolgirl in the land would envy us our opportunities, which cannot have been true. The only other sea I knew was the Atlantic Ocean which was the other side of Ireland; in addition to being cold, it had huge breakers, and if you did ever manage to get into it, people were always running out after you to try and save you. But the Mediterranean was and is beautiful, blue and warm. I saw it not from a yacht or a villa, but from the deck of a very poor-grade ship where students used to lie in sleeping bags way back in the 1960s, when we were all discovering the world. I used to sit up in my sleeping bag, even at night, and watch it rolling by the ship. I knew I'd never see as marvellous a sea again, and I never did.

My third wonder was the discovery of Welsh male voice choirs. For no reason at all the sound got me right at the back of the throat the first time I heard one, and a choir can still do it today. I can't understand what they're singing, and it's not my religion or culture or nation, but when they go into all that easy harmony and swirling and soaring I feel somehow as if they're my tribe, and tears will trickle down my face as I listen to Welshmen singing. It happens at ridiculous places like Cardiff Arms Park at the Wales *v.* Ireland rugby international, or when I was doing a story about the miners' strike.

Another wonder came to me through work. I was a teacher once, and worked for eight years in girls' schools. People who are still at school will probably find this pathetic, but there is almost no wonder compared with the realization that a child has actually understood something. I know that this could sound defeatist and cynical – after all, the children are meant to understand what the teacher teaches them: that's the system. But it doesn't actually happen all that often – that lovely dawning, the 'I *see*!' which is music to the ears. And no Mr Chips or Miss Jean Brodie could ever have been as happy as I was on the rare occasions when a girl would suddenly discover the pleasure of poetry, and see that people read it because they liked it, and because it sounded rhythmic and exciting.

My fifth choice is something that one has grown oneself. I usually only have to look at a plant and it dies. Friends have fronds and trailing greenery all over their houses, but even the busiest of Lizzies will turn to decay in my hands. But the summer I grew tomatoes was the start of a new wonder. I watched them nervously from pea-sized and pea-green colour until they became big, glorious, red and ripe. I used to dream about them and hurry home from work to see if they were still alive. I apologized in my mind to people for ever having thought them gardening bores, and I used to sit and listen to *Gardeners' Question Time* with my ear right up to the set.

It sounds self-centred to say that I love hearing people agreeing with something I wrote, but it sometimes takes a lot of courage to put your own thoughts out there, in case other people will say you're silly. Occasionally, though not very often, I hear people say, 'I agree with that woman utterly.' Or if they've been to a play of mine they might say, 'I know exactly what she means. I know someone just like that.' It is a wonder to me that for years and years I wanted to be a writer, and now I am. But it's just as bad each time you write something – the anxiety about whether people will like it is just as great.

It's a very big wonder – perhaps the biggest – to have someone to welcome you back from places. When I was young and used to roam the world on a student's grant and then on an impoverished teacher's earnings, much of the pleasure was in coming home and telling it all to a family that was so interested and who cared about every move. I remember my father getting out an atlas, and my mother used to look over all the postcards I'd sent and check what adventure had happened in each place. And now, too, when I come home from a business trip or even a very exhausting day, the whole thing seems to fall into place properly because of the welcome and the interest and the fact that someone knows and wants to know about what you did. Perhaps it's because I love talking so much, but I would find coming back to an empty house very flat and pointless. Some of my friends and colleagues say that they love the freedom and the peace and the independence of getting back from somewhere to silence, and being able to take off their shoes and say nothing and do nothing. But I'd find it far from wonderful to come back just to four walls.

Writer and broadcaster John Julius Norwich appears frequently on television and among his many other activities is chairman of the Venice in Peril fund

There were three periods in my life when travelling by train was really exciting. One was when I was a small boy, just before the war, and my mother used to take me twice a year to France, and occasionally even to Italy. That involved going on the night sleeper, and for a boy of seven going on the night sleeper and charging through the night past all sorts of strange wayside stations was marvellous. Later, after the war, when we lived in France, I used to go backwards and forwards a lot on the night ferry, which had its own special charm. The train actually went on to the boat, and I would wake up in the middle of the night when it was probably cold and wet and, with any luck, snowing. I would hear all these people working to get the train on to the boat and then off again, and chains clanking and voices yelling, and occasionally awful muffled oaths when they dropped a chain on their foot. I loved the thought of all these wonderful people working hard for me in conditions of extreme discomfort, while I was lying tucked up cosily in bed. Much later I worked at the British Embassy in Belgrade, possibly the last European capital without aeroplanes, so one had to travel by the Orient Express every time and that was straight out of an Eric Ambler thriller.

Number two is caviar, to me a great proof of the generosity and lavishness of nature. I like the idea of fish laying millions and millions and millions of eggs, of which two hatch out. All the others are totally wasted, except those in the form of caviar, which I can eat. It's the most perfect taste experience known to man, and the marvellous thing is that it should be a raw material. God is still one up on humanity – with all the great cooking that the world has achieved, caviar is nevertheless just that little bit better. But the one thing it's got to have is quantity, and of course that's the one thing it very seldom does have. There's no point buying a little two-ounce pot – you've got to have it by the quarter pound at least, and eat it, if possible, with a silver shoehorn.

My third one is the Taj Mahal. Hackneyed, you may say, and indeed it is. Why does the Taj Mahal have to be the most beautiful building in the world? Wouldn't it be lovely if one could find some other building that nobody knew about, that everybody didn't agree was the most beautiful? But there it is, you can't. You go to the Taj Mahal and it's game, set and match from the moment you first see the thing. It wins every time. Nothing can stand behind it because there's a gigantic river far lower than it. It stands there etched against the sky, white, and with those very deep windows – great darknesses. So there's always this marvellous play of sunshine and shadow, and that and the purity, the contrast between strength and delicacy, between the straight lines and the curves, the dark and the light, all takes your breath away.

I suppose we all love sunshine, but nothing else has for me such power of total transformation. It's the combination of the physical pleasure of warmth, and the way the colours and shapes of things suddenly come out in a way they never have before. And other people come out, too. Everybody's nicer in the sunshine; everybody says: 'Isn't it a lovely day?' and smiles. The sunshine doesn't necessarily need to be undiluted. It can be the kind of effect you get in Ireland, with lovely shafts of watery light suddenly illuminating a green hill where everything else is in darkness. Or that wonderful sunshine against a black, thundery sky when a little white church, say, is picked out and made luminous against this background.

Wine, like caviar, is to me certain proof of the existence of God. It's so marvellous that the juice of the grape should metamorphose in this miraculous way; if you leave orange juice, it just stays orange juice. It always seems to me that one of the nicest of all miracles, the Marriage at Cana, really did a lot of good. I discovered the other day that the Bible actually tells you how much water was transformed into wine, and by our present measures it comes to about nine hundred bottles. And that was only after they had finished the first lot. It really must have been quite a party. Incidentally, I'm not a connoisseur of wine. I just like enormous quantities of plonk – Château Filthy every time, in great flowing beakers.

Chess – I can't play it, or hardly; I have practically never won a game in my life, but I see its incredible majesty. I see that it's the king of games. I don't think it necessarily reveals intelligence, but it does reveal a power of understanding mathematical beauty and the ability to subordinate the great universal logic to one's own will. Seeing the pleasure of building up these grand designs of enormous complexity, and then seeing the whole thing fit neatly into place, must be one of the most glorious and powerful feelings the human spirit is capable of.

Finally my own great love – the city of Venice, to me another great miracle. It is a city built in the most unpromising site conceivable. Who on earth would want to go to a lot of soggy, shallow shoals and sandbanks in the middle of a malarial lagoon in the fifth century? But there it is – they did. In fact it was originally a funk hole for people fleeing from the Barbarians. They built not just a city but an incredibly beautiful city, this magical thing which is totally unlike any other in the world and which, because of that water, has been protected from everything all

51

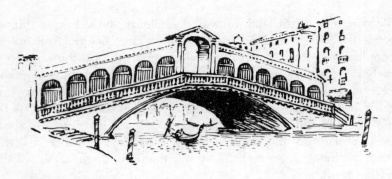

through history. It's never been destroyed, pillaged or invaded – the only great Italian city that hasn't suffered such a fate. Above all, nowadays, it's the one city which has been protected from the greatest scourge of the twentieth century, the motor car. In this marvellous place where everybody goes everywhere by boat or on foot not only is it beautiful, but life is gentler, quieter, easier; nobody has heart attacks, strokes or high blood pressure – all you get is rheumatism, and it's worth it every time.

Author and broadcaster Arthur Marshall

The personal wonders that have brightened my life are many and varied, and high on the list – and how happy I am to be able at last to give it a public word of thanks – is my hot water bottle. No possession that has come my way on Life's Highroad has ever given me greater satisfaction. It hasn't, of course, always been the same hot water bottle. Hot water bottles come and go, or rather, they come and leak and go. I'm breaking in a new one at the moment – delicately ribbed and in a rather striking shade of pink, and already a real pal. It warms up my pyjamas before I climb into them, and then it gets busy warming outlying portions of me. And there's another advantage. Waking in the night, I just stick out a toe and the bottle's heat, or reduced heat, tells me just where we are – 2.40, 4.15, or 6.50, with dawn over the horizon. Some people enshroud their bottles in covers. Not me. I like them naked and unashamed and giving off their full rich and rubbery aroma.

Another never-failing wonder to me is that dish called bubble and squeak. Some people seem never to have heard of it and give nervous cries of 'Whatever's this?', and I have astonished many a guest with my culinary expertise. Whoever would have thought that leftover bits of cooked vegetables – spuds, cauli, cabbage, carrots – all rough-cut and pressed together into a flat round cake and then vigorously fried on both sides, would transform themselves into such a poem of crisp deliciousness. Good heavens, I'm dribbling at the very thought.

To get away for a moment from creature comforts, I confess to an undying admiration for Her Majesty's Theatre in London, a glory, when I first saw it in 1917, of red velvet and cream and gold. It was my first London theatre, and *Chu Chin Chow* was on, and twelve years later there was *Bitter Sweet* and what more could a stage-struck person ask for? During the Blitz in the war, one vaguely wondered where the bomb with one's name on it would get one, and I always hoped that, if Her Majesty's had to go, I would be there too, preferably at the end of a performance – too irritating to be struck down during the overture.

Do you smell something? There's a funny whiff in the air, as unforgettable and unforgotten as Rupert Brooke's Grantchester river smell, and it means, for this is a country smell too, that somebody somewhere has got a bonfire. Oh, the pleasure of collecting the combustibles, lighting them, stoking them, poking them and, after assuming that they are finally dead, suddenly seeing that little wisp of smoke curling up. As with bubble and squeak, who could believe that such a wonder would come from base and unwanted materials, and with, later, the splendour of bonfire ash to scatter here and there in the garden.

And then there's my portable gramophone, a permanent pleasure, although I really prefer those gramophones that you have to wind up by hand so that you feel you have somehow earned the record. But they don't seem to make them any more and so mine is an early electric one and real joy, for I only play those old records called 78s and the machine makes the sort of loud and fairly tinny sound that suits so well many of the dear old tunes – 'Swanee' and 'Dolly Gray' and 'Any Time's Kissing Time'. I'm also extremely partial to 'The Laughing Policeman', but I do see that it's rather an acquired taste.

There are just so many more wonders. The virtually deserted City of London at night or in the early morning. The smell of freshly baked bread. The sight of witch-hazel glowing away on the darkest winter day. The crackle of dead leaves. Sunrise and sunset. And have you noticed something about the wonders I have mentioned? Most of them either cost very little, or nothing at all.

A SPECIMEN DAY

Lady Stevens

It was with a sense of wondering relief that I pulled the bedclothes up to my chin and stretched out for my hot milk and book, and settled to read. It was a Thursday night in March, and as I read Quentin Bell's biography of his aunt, Virginia Woolf, I came to a paragraph in which she had described one of her 'specimen' days. 'How strange,' I thought, 'a good way to describe today', and my mind went back to eleven o'clock that morning.

It was warm, with the first smell of spring in the air. Letters to solicitors and cheques had been dealt with dutifully before I stepped outside to join Dobson, the gardener, who was pruning roses.

'Good morning, Dobson. What a glorious day.'

'Yes', he replied, and then there was a short silence before he added: 'There is water leaking from the manhole.'

We prised open the lid with a garden spade and he was right; it was full and blocked. There are three manholes in the garden, covering an independent sewage system. Each revealed worse horrors. I peered down the last black hole and saw below unspeakable sludge covered with red worms, writhing slowly. As I pushed around with an old axe handle the stench was nose-choking and I imagined the horror of falling in. Would Dobson haul me out, or panic and leave me? And if I could get out, would I spend the rest of my life with a morbid obsession about never being able to get my skin clean, however much I washed?

The nightmare passed in a flash as I called for buckets and a large garden sieve. We placed the sieve over the sludge hole and tipped buckets full of mixture from the two blocked holes through the sieve in order to retrieve the offending yards of lavatory paper. This operation lasted two hours, while Dobson, with averted eyes, attended carefully to his roses.

Feeling a certain sense of triumph I asked him to turn on the hose, and I sprayed everything over and over until all the tools and my feet were soaked. Now for a bath. But this was not to be, for Dobson couldn't turn off the hose tap – the washer had gone. I ran down to the cellar and turned the water off at the mains. It was a stroke of unexpected good luck that I caught the plumber at home. It was lunch-time. He promised to come quickly, but he was delayed an hour and a half. That evening I had four friends coming for dinner and nothing was ready. By about four o'clock the tap was mended and I bathed and washed my hair; I felt grateful to be clean again.

The meal had been arranged as a prelude to an ecumenical Lenten discussion in our church, which is next door to my home. My friends and I were the last in, and the vicar commented that the Roman Catholics were more punctual. As the churchwarden stood up to give an introductory talk on individual prayer my neighbour nudged me.

'Jane, isn't that your cat?' she asked, pointing to a black tail moving along the front pew.

It certainly was my cat, but I looked intently at the speaker. Snuffs got bored with pew-walking and took to the aisle, gazing with interest at those seated near to him and obviously looking for me. A man behind grabbed him and put him outside the church door. The speaker continued, urging us to greater concentration when praying. Challenging his voice came another from outside – a loud and determined yowl that could only belong to a Siamese, my Siamese. The churchwarden soldiered on to the end.

We were split up into groups by the vicar for more personal discussion. Without warning he turned to me and said: 'Jane, will you please give the summing-up for your group?' This was the end. Now I should be unable to leave the church to take my cat home. Fortunately a Roman Catholic in our group gave her views on the virtue of prayer through the rosary, and then changed the subject quickly, saying, 'Wouldn't your cat be happier inside?' Thankfully I assured her that all he wanted was a warm lap and some firm stroking. He adores making a scene and had embarrassed me many times in the past. He would stalk me at a distance when I was going out to dinner in the village, and then yowl outside the house until he was allowed to join in the feast.

'And how do you feel about prayer?' I asked a member of the

group in a desperately serious voice. By this time Snuffs had achieved his aim and was looking smug. With two others I gave an outwardly calm and measured report on the thoughts of our group. Beneath was an urgent need to escape and I grabbed the cat and almost ran out of the church. But that was not the end of the day's events. As I opened the front door, dropped the cat, and rushed into the sitting-room to check on my dog, Sophy, I forgot the second alarm key. A penetrating, clanging alarm bell started up. In church the vicar was taking Compline, a service designed to form a peaceful ending to a discussion such as we had just had. I fought with the bunch of keys, found the right one, and at last, with trembling hand, I turned it in the lock, quieting the bell.

So ended a day which could fairly be called a 'specimen'. I don't mind them, but hope that in the others that must surely follow the subject matter will be widely different.

BELOW STAIRS

Adeline Hartcup has studied the archives of seven great houses, discovering how the servants lived during the nineteenth century*

The largest staff list that I found was that of the Duke of Bridgwater, who had five hundred servants. At the beginning of this century, when times were bad and a lot of his tenants were out of work, he increased his staff list to eight hundred just to help things. People tend to forget that the owners of these huge houses were great employers, and quite paternalistic. They were good educators. They also looked after their servants' morals, and saw that the valets – and indeed their own sons – didn't come near the housemaids' bedrooms. I found evidence of this when I was looking through the archives. When one of the sons of the house began to grow up and take an interest in a pretty housemaid, the maid tended to be spirited away to the dairy or one of the home farms.

Lady Frederick Cavendish had difficulties with her lady's maids. She said that, in spite of prayer, she somehow never managed to appoint the right one. She was upset by this and said: 'I'm so tired of having these grumpy, difficult lady's maids. At last I've got a paragon, Mrs Parry, and now all is going to be plain sailing.' But it's rather a sad story because shortly afterwards there's a note in the records saying: 'Mrs Parry seemed perfect, but after a month she told me she was pregnant', and she was pregnant with 'a luckless baby' as she put it. And that was the end of Mrs Parry.

Sometimes the servants weren't terribly happy with their employers, of course. There were two cases in particular. The Duke of Cumberland, the son of George III, was a very disagreeable character, and his valet attacked and nearly murdered him. And at Woburn Lord William Russell did get murdered by his Swiss manservant, who seized a knife from the sideboard and cut his throat. What must have happened more often, though, was servants displeasing their master or mistress and being sent off without a reference, when of course it would be very hard to get another job.

Etiquette in the servants' hall was almost as rigid as it was above stairs. The servants were divided into upper servants and under servants. Sometimes they dined in completely separate rooms. At Longleat the upper servants would proceed into the servants' hall arm-in-arm, very stately and formal, and would take the first part of the meal with the under servants. Then, after the roast, they would stand up and proceed equally ceremoniously to the housekeeper's room, where they would have wine and coffee and their pudding and refined conversation.

Many of these houses weren't occupied for more than about two months of the year by the family, and a few servants moved around with them. Obviously the lady's maid and the valet would move, because they accompanied their master and mistress wherever they went, and the housekeeper sometimes went, and one or two of the top housemaids and top livery men. The others stayed behind, but there must have been a great deal of upkeep in these enormous houses and there were many jobs that could only be done when the family was away from home.

Spring cleaning was a terrific game and it gives one an inferiority complex to hear about it, though one must also feel thankful. The curtains were all brought down and the carpets were taken up. The old polish was washed off the furniture with vinegar and replaced with generous coatings of beeswax and turpentine; then the wood was rubbed until it was warm and gleamed again. In these very high rooms the servants had to stand on long ladders to wash the ceilings with soda and water. They cleaned the paint-work and then polished it with a cream dressing. Something called linen drugget, which some of us can just remember, was draped along the picture rails. Venetian blinds were an awful lot of work – they were scrubbed on both sides and then strung up again. At Longleat the furniture was scoured and calendered. Scouring meant polishing the metal or wood surfaces with fine sand, or rubbing the cloth with soap, and calendering meant pressing the cloth or paper in a calender, which is a device fitted with rollers to smooth or glaze wrinkled materials.

The corridors were cleaned and whitened with fine pipeclay. While this was being done, sheets of drugget were spread over the carpets. The brocades on the walls were a very difficult task: they were dusted down with soft brushes, then rubbed over, first of all with tissue paper and later with very soft silk dusters. The floors were washed and then anointed with beeswax and turpentine; this was left to dry and finally a shiny surface was produced by pushing a huge, lead-weighted polisher up and down. This machine was also used before a ball, when the floor was sprinkled with French chalk to make it slippery.

Were the servants happy in those days? I think so, on the whole, because life was very hard outside the park gates, and families were large and overcrowded. If you got into one of the great houses you had to leave your home, and up to a point you gave up quite a lot of freedom, but you got four good meals a day – the servants usually had two roasts every day, which is far more than most of us get today – and rations of beer with lunch and supper. They also got their clothes, they had a roof over their heads, and, what was probably more valuable than anything else, they had a training. In those days a village girl had a pretty scanty chance of a training anywhere else. Which of these houses would I have chosen to work in as a servant? That's a difficult question. I think I'd have preferred to be a duchess in one of them!

*Her book based on these researches, *Below Stairs in the Great Country Houses*, is published by Sidgwick and Jackson

CHOOSING AND CARING FOR BEDDING AND BEDCLOTHES

Muriel Clark is a home economist

It's quite surprising that to equip a bed with conventional blankets costs just about the same as equipping it with a continental quilt, so if you're starting off and trying to make a choice, there isn't much in it financially, and continental quilts do save a lot of work. What's inside them? The most expensive quilts are filled with plumage – waterfowl plumage, which as a rule is duck or eider-duck down; the latter is the most expensive of all. It has a very high tog rating, which is the latest way of measuring the amount of warmth which you can expect from a quilt. The higher the number, the warmer the quilt should be – a tog rating of 11.5, for example, would relate to a plumage quilt, and would mean that you'd get a lot of warmth. But a high tog rating can also mean a lot of weight, so when you're buying look at the tog rating alongside the weight of the quilt, and think what it will be like to sleep under.

The second most expensive type of filling is down and feather, and then there is feather and down (whichever material is named first is in a higher proportion). The cheapest of the lot are polyester fillings, which have been improved tremendously over recent years. Research has given us much lighter-weight polyester fillings which stay in place – in the past they tended to go lumpy – and these are ideal for anyone with an allergy. They are also good for children's and invalids' beds because they are washable.

I wouldn't, however, recommend putting a washable quilt in your own washing machine. If you can, take it to a launderette, which is the best place to wash them. All the other sorts of fillings need dry cleaning, but if you look after them properly they should last for about twenty years without cleaning. Have a good cover which you wash regularly, and if anything gets spilt on the quilt whip the top cover off quickly and push the filling away from the part where the spill is, so that you can sponge or wash that bit of the cover. It's very important to air a continental quilt – if you've been on holiday in Europe you will probably have seen them hanging out on the balconies. Air it regularly near an open window, because the body can lose a third of a litre of moisture during the night and it's all got to go somewhere, so some of it must end up in the quilt. If there are two people in the bed a quilt can in fact become quite damp.

Blankets are made today in a variety of fibres, though wool is still the traditional one. It is also the most expensive, and needs some care in washing. King-size blankets are too big for a domestic machine and are best taken to a launderette. Wool is best washed in a mild product at a low temperature, with minimum agitation; automatic machines will be suitably programmed. It is important to observe any drying instructions on the care label, too, especially regarding tumble driers. Acrylic fibre blankets should be washed and dried in the same way, as high temperatures may cause stretching. Cotton cellular blankets are the easiest of all to wash and sterilize, so they are ideal for children and invalids; their cellular structure provides the warmth.

Pillow fillings are very much the same as continental quilt ones. Again, anyone with an allergy will want a polyester-filled pillow. The foam rubber ones have gone out of fashion, and they were rather hot. One of the most interesting developments I've seen recently is a new, non-woven 'pillow protector', which looks rather like paper and is made out of polyester fibres. You put that on your pillow under the normal pillow case and it stops any moisture going through, so that the pillow underneath doesn't get stained. They're quite expensive, costing about as much as a conventional pillow case, but they can be washed, they last for a long time, and they do protect your pillows. I've been experimenting with one for a manufacturer for some time, and I'm very impressed with it.

Polyester and cotton fabric seems to be the in-thing for sheets today, but it does have an affinity for grease, and people's greasy skins, face cream and hair oil can stain your pillows and bed linen quite badly. You must wash polyester and cotton really frequently, more often than old-fashioned linen and cotton, and use a solvent detergent if possible, because that helps get rid of the greasiness. Deeper colours and patterns, of course, don't show the soiling, but remember that they do get soiled just as quickly and will still need regular washing. A fitted sheet, although it makes bedmaking much easier, is less flexible than a flat one. If you have an unexpected guest and you've only got two fitted sheets available, you've got a problem. Finally, you can't sides-to-middle a fitted sheet, of course. And with the price of bed linen today, I think we might be sides-to-middling more often than in the past few years.

CREME CARAMEL

Mary Berry's recipe serves four people

Caramel
3 oz (90 g) granulated sugar
3 tablespoons water

Custard
4 eggs
1½ oz (40 g) caster sugar
few drops of vanilla essence
1 pint (600 ml) milk

Pre-heat the oven to 300°F (150°C, gas mark 2). To make the caramel put the sugar and water in a heavy saucepan and dissolve the sugar over a low heat. Bring to the boil, and continue boiling until the syrup is a pale golden brown. Remove from the heat and quickly pour the caramel into a 1½ pint (900 ml) charlotte mould, cake tin or soufflé dish. Allow to cool.

For the custard, mix together the eggs, sugar and vanilla essence. Warm the milk in a saucepan over a low heat until it is hand-hot, then pour it on to the egg mixture, stirring constantly. Butter the sides of the mould above the caramel. Strain the custard into the mould and place in a roasting tin half filled with water. Bake for 1½ hours or until a knife inserted in the centre comes out clean. Don't worry if it takes longer to cook than the time given – it will set eventually. Do not increase the oven temperature, or the custard will have bubbles in it. Remove from the oven and leave to cool completely for at least 12 hours or overnight. Turn out carefully on to a flat dish deep enough to catch the caramel juices.

MARY BURCHELL

The President of the Romantic Novelists' Association talks about her long and fascinating life, and in particular her love of opera

The two great passions in my life are opera and writing, and the second really stemmed from the first. My sister Louise and I had our first great adventure when we were young office girls in the 1920s: we decided to save up and go to America to hear the great Galli-Curci singing opera. It took us a long time, but we managed it, and as a result I wrote my first article. Then I got the offer of a small job in Fleet Street, as a fiction sub-editress at 4 guineas a week – I thought I'd hit the jackpot! While there, I was encouraged by my editress to write fiction, and so I wrote my first romantic novel, *Wife to Christopher*. If we had not gone to America to hear opera none of it would have happened.

I think we were so determined to go to America – which was really quite adventurous for young girls in those days – because Galli-Curci's was the first voice we fell in love with. We heard her in concert here in Britain and knew we just had to hear her sing in opera. After I had made some inquiries and discovered that she sang opera only in New York, it was to New York that we had to go; we'd never even been alone to Brighton for the day when we made this decision. So we set to work. I was earning £2 10s a week – £2.50 in modern terms; Louise was earning just a little more. We decided we could do the whole thing on £100 each – those were the happy days when you could go to New York and back for £36 10s, third-class tourist. We went by ship, of course, for there were no aeroplanes then. That first article, incidentally, written as a result of this trip, was about the clothes that we had made to take with us. In those days everyone made their own clothes. We took our patterns from a magazine called *Mab's Fashions* – there was a free pattern every month, and the others were a shilling each, as I recall.

We thought we must tell one person about this extraordinary idea of ours, and so I wrote to Galli-Curci to tell her we were coming. She wrote back saying, 'If you ever succeed in getting to America, you shall have tickets for everything I sing.' And indeed she was as good as her word. When we eventually got to America, there we were with seats for everything, and even met Galli-Curci herself. It was the first of our great operatic adventures. I suppose it was surprising that somebody so famous should have taken so much trouble to look after us, but even then I always believed in a happy ending as long as one had worked for it. It seemed fantastic, gorgeous . . . but not impossible. I always felt that if you know what you want, and are prepared to do the right things to get it, the chances are that, though you won't necessarily get what you are after, something marvellous will come out of it. It certainly did for me.

Something very different, but also brought about by opera, happened in the 1930s, when we were able to help Jews and other refugees escape from Hitler's Germany. It all started when Louise and I went to the Salzburg Musical Festival in Austria in 1934. Some of our operatic darlings were performing there, and among them were the great Viennese conductor Clemens Krauss and his wife, who was a famous singer. We didn't know them, but we stood at the stage door and said, 'Wonderful performance to-night', which is what opera fans do. In those days everything was very pleasant and informal, and they were very kind to us and introduced us to the official lecturer, who was a great friend of theirs. They explained that she would be coming to London later in the year, and asked if we would look after her. We didn't know why she wanted looking after, since she looked much better able to look after herself than we did, but we were flattered.

In due course we found ourselves showing her all the sights. When we went to Westminster Abbey she asked, 'Is this Protestant or Catholic?' We told her. Then we went to St Paul's and again she asked, 'Is this Protestant or Catholic?'

I thought perhaps I should ask which she was, and so – under the dome of St Paul's, I remember – I inquired, 'Which are you, Protestant or Catholic?'

'Didn't you know?' she replied, 'I'm a Jewess.'

We weren't even interested. We were so green then that we didn't know that to be Jewish and to come from Frankfurt-am-Main in Germany, as she did, already had the seeds of tragedy in it. But she stayed quite a while, and we got to know her very well. Through her eyes, and the eyes of a Jewish family in Germany, we began to see what was going on. And so we started to help this family to get out. At that moment, for the first time in my life, I began to make money, and that enabled me to be of assistance to them and to others. We went on until the week before war broke out, and we got twenty-nine people out altogether.

We also smuggled out their furs and jewellery and other valuables, and that was where being a fiction writer was very helpful, because I could talk my way out of almost anything. We still had to be very careful, though. We never took ear-rings for pierced ears, for instance, since we didn't have pierced ears. That was the sort of thing the German police caught you on. You had to know how people tick, and how far you could go. It was rather dangerous, but less so than it might sound.

Our cover story was always that we were two very naive opera fans, coming to Germany to hear opera. Clemens Krauss, who was really the instigator of it all, was director of the Munich Opera in those days, and helped us immeasurably. When we told him we were getting nervous he hit on a perfectly simple plan. Each time, before we left, we were to tell him what days we wanted covered, and he would tell us what he would put on at the opera house on those nights. He sent us back fully primed, so that to the Germans we seemed just like starry-eyed opera fans coming from a special performance. He never let us down once, and under cover of what must have been some of the greatest operatic performances of the century we did our work. We remained in contact with all twenty-nine of our escapees, though in the natural course of events some of them have since died. But Else Mayer-Lismann, the daughter of the first woman we got out, the official lecturer in Salzburg whom we entertained in London, became official lecturer at Glyndebourne and Edinburgh, and now she's like another sister to us.

In time we got to know personally a number of great names in the opera world, and I even ghosted Tito Gobbi's autobiography. That was an opera fan's dream, of course. If someone had come to me when I was a girl, standing in the queue at Covent Garden, and said that one day I would help to write the life story of a schoolboy in Italy destined to become one of the greatest operatic artists of the century, I'd have thought they were talking nonsense.

I don't find opera and romantic fiction an awkward combination. I'm not really a compulsive writer, but I enjoy doing it, and trying to do it well. I'm sure I could have been perfectly happy doing something else, provided I still got the same enjoyment out of life. I've written some 160 books and certainly don't remember them all, but I sometimes go back and read them. I do love them, and as soon as I've started I will recall the central characters, but a group of interesting cousins or something like that I will read about with passionate curiosity, as if I had not invented them in the first place. Opera comes into my novels – in particular the conductor Oscar Warrender who has appeared in more recent books. Everybody's in love with him, including me. One day somebody wrote me a charming letter saying, 'Don't you think it's time he was knighted?' I wrote back saying it was a wonderful idea, and knighted him forthwith.

Although I've never married, I don't find it difficult to write about my heroines when they are passionately in love. Everybody has had some real or vicarious romance in their lives. I certainly know how young people react to it, and the interesting thing is that they don't change through the generations. I remember rather well how I was as a girl, and also what scared me, which is very important. I suppose that the heroine always in some sense reflects the writer and, 'my girl' is various forms of myself. I love working out how people respond to each other, and in this connection all one's experience of people becomes very important.

I've been lucky enough to share a house with my sister Louise all my life. Although I handle the business side of my work myself she is really the more studious one, while I'm the bossy one. We do, however, work marvellously together, mostly because she's totally devoid of jealousy. If there are two of you, and one of you has a little success, it's not easy to be the other one, but Louise has never been anything but happy with me.

DR HELENA WRIGHT

Now a lively lady in her nineties, Dr Wright was one of the pioneers of the family planning movement in Britain and knew Marie Stopes well

Fifty years ago, when the three family planning clinics in London and one or two outside London all joined together to form one, solid movement, we were dealing only with married women, and even special kinds of married women – only working-class women who really had more children than they wanted. In those days there was not only total ignorance about sex, but also total disbelief. An idea such as limiting the number of children they had had never occurred to them. You might just as well have said, 'If you go out in the rain, we'll tell you how to stop it raining.' They were very honest people, and they had to discover for themselves that we were telling the truth. They also had to grow in self-confidence, so that they could carry out what they were being taught.

My background is a mixed one. My father was Polish, from a land-owning family in the corner of Poland which used to belong to Austria. My mother was British – as British as she could be – and they made a marvellous couple because they were so different. We went to the family estate in Poland every other summer, and all the cousins met. Between us we represented three nations – Polish, German and British – which was very good for us. I don't really speak Polish any more. German I can get away with, though, as long as the other person isn't too abstruse.

I was at medical school just before the First World War, from 1910 to 1914. There were thirteen other women in my year, and we were all definitely rather odd. But as we were all together we didn't think about the fact that we were women among so many men. We were there because we wished to be there, and to work. We had a very good, extremely constructive set of teachers, and a reasonable curriculum.

I knew Marie Stopes, perhaps the best-known pioneer of birth control, very well. In a curious way our paths coincided. In 1918, when my husband and I were in Cornwall with our first baby, she and her second husband turned up at the same hotel. The two husbands liked each other very much, and the two wives also liked each other. A lot of people found her rather frightening, but I thought she was very alive and full of ideas and purpose. My interest in family planning came about through my training as a doctor and subsequently as a gynaecologist, and not because of any influence from Marie Stopes. She was a perfectly genuine scientist, the first woman MSc in London University, and an expert on fossil coal, but she was not a doctor. She had her own purpose – she wished to help her fellow women in any situation in which they felt themselves degraded or in peril or over-awed. In 1930 I insisted that my fellow family planning helpers let her join us.

At this time, when birth control work was just starting in

Britain, the seeds of an international movement had been sown. However the people that we joined up with in Britain had their gaze only on this country, and I had to keep quiet – I was the only one who was conscious that we were taking part in a movement in which three other countries, the United States, Sweden and Holland, were involved in the same private way. In all these countries there were central pioneer personalities, to whom the rest of the workers were indebted. We didn't really compare notes at all, though I met them when I was travelling abroad.

The early methods – and we had to invent a number of them – were the barrier ones, which couldn't have been simpler: a natural, mechanical barrier inside the woman, plus a kind of harmless chemical which saw to it that all the sperm of any one intercourse died before there was a chance of their getting past at all. So simple, so obvious; and it's still the best method because it can't fail.

By the time of the outbreak of the Second World War we were fairly well established, but we were dependent on rubber, because all the caps were made of that material – and all the rubber was needed for the war. We looked about and found, through great good luck, that a very big rubber company had had a huge order from Paris for some hotel bathroom floors. So sheets and sheets of coloured rubber were offered to us; we said thank you very much. It made excellent caps, which became heirlooms in the families of the people who had them. When I was still working, which was about eight years ago, very occasionally someone would come up and say, 'I've still got my "Helena".' They used to call them Helenas for fun!

We got no support at all from the medical schools, incidentally, during the 1930s. Fairly soon after we were established, when we realized that this must be a national piece of work, our Secretary wrote personally to the deans of all the medical schools in London. Not one of them answered.

The second stage in our pioneering efforts was a perfectly logical one – to deal with married women before their first pregnancy, so that they would start their marriage knowing that they could plan their own family. That was very important, because our first steps had been negative ones, whereas this was definitely positive. We encouraged mothers to bring their daughters to us generally two or three weeks before they were married. This development had interesting beginnings. At one of the sessions in North Kensington where I worked for thirty years, one of my old patients approached me and said she wished to ask something rather special. She told me that her eldest daughter was engaged. Then she looked at me and said, 'Is it possible for you to teach her, before she's married, what you've taught me so successfully?' That was the beginning of that stage of the movement; vision among the patients was very important. We started helping unmarried girls very much later – I've forgotten the date, but there was a great national controversy.

I still feel that my life's work is in mid-career, though I stopped working in general practice when I was eighty-five, which I thought was time enough. I have had a very happy marriage, with four failures and four sons; we always wanted daughters, though, but we couldn't face a possible fifth son. Luckily among the grandchildren there's one girl; her father and mother are both doctors, so it was almost inevitable that she should choose medicine as a career. She's now a student at the Royal Free Hospital, which was my old hospital. Exactly seventy years separated my arrival there and hers.

SHEILA KITZINGER

Something of a guru for many women because of her views on pregnancy and childbirth, Sheila Kitzinger has written several books, is on the advisory board of the National Childbirth Trust, and feels that doctors and hospitals tend to be too rigid in their views on how women should give birth

It was my training as a social anthropolgist that led me to my work with pregnancy and childbirth. When I first became pregnant myself, I discovered that we really didn't know much about how women felt and behaved in different countries. All the anthropological work had been done almost exclusively by men, and they hadn't asked questions about birth; there was a big literature on what was done to the placenta, because they had stood outside the birth huts of primitive tribes and had seen that happening, but they didn't really know what went on inside. So I became very interested in what it felt like to be a woman giving birth in different societies, which of course included our own.

When my youngest child was about two and a half I took the whole family to Jamaica, where I studied West Indian peasant women and urban poor. One of the important things that I noticed was that women didn't spontaneously lie down to have a baby. Whenever possible they kept moving around, right through the first stage of labour; and indeed even in the second stage, if they could get into an upright or semi-upright position, they did. In fact if a West Indian woman had a chance she would rock her pelvis in a kind of belly-dancing movement, very similar to the movements that women engage in in the Revivalist Churches, when they're getting the spirit and going to speak with tongues. Their whole approach to labour is that it's something the mother does for herself, and that she should be mobile and active; she doesn't just lie there passively, having something done to her. The midwives in the hospitals didn't like this attitude, because they thought the women ought to lie down and be good patients.

In Britain enormous changes have been made over the last two or three years. We have now discovered – and there's been plenty of research work to support this – that it's much safer for a woman to have at least the upper part of her body well raised, or even to be standing, for much of labour. The uterus contracts better, the woman feels less pain, and the baby is better oxygenated. First of all this was looked at in terms of the first stage of labour, and then also in terms of the second stage. No woman in her right mind would choose to lie down on her back with her legs in the air to push a baby out, because she has to push uphill. Most women, if allowed to do what they want to do, and what comes naturally, will adopt a modified squatting position, crouch or kneel forward, or even get on all fours. Hospitals are now beginning to see that they achieve more effective second stages if they encourage women to adopt any position which is comfortable for them. I think this is marvellous – it means we have to do away with the old-fashioned delivery room beds, and put mattresses on the floor and provide lots of pillows and something more like the medieval birthing stool – a very low, horseshoe-shaped kind of milking stool – which women right through history used to sit on to have babies.

All this, of course, challenges the current preference in hospitals generally for mechanized, monitored birth. But what is the point of rupturing the membranes, inserting an electrode and putting a clip on to a baby's scalp, and having a woman lying down and monitoring every heartbeat, if you are thereby producing a dip in the foetal heartbeat? There is also plenty of evidence to suggest that having a woman immobile, and rupturing the membranes artificially, thus taking away the protective bubble of water in which the baby is lying, actually produce the conditions which we then go on and monitor.

One of the reasons put forward by doctors for this controlled form of giving birth is to reduce perinatal mortality. In fact Britain has rather a low perinatal mortality rate, though it is going down more slowly than in some parts of Europe and certainly than in Japan. Of course babies are precious and we don't want them to die unnecessarily, but sometimes I hear a doctor say that the one thing that matters is a live and healthy baby – quite honestly, for most families it *isn't* the only thing that matters. The way one feels about that baby, and the bonds that link you with it, are important too, and there's really no point in producing a perfect, well-oxygenated, healthy little animal unless the relationship between the baby and its parents is a going concern. That's why I think we have to look at the whole culture of childbirth in our society and see what we can do to make it a celebration, a joyous occasion.

My own approach to giving birth I describe as 'psycho-sexual', a term I use because I think birth is essentially a sexual activity. By this I mean not only that sex starts the baby off, but that the rhythms of birth are essentially sexual, if we allow them to be. I suspect that most of our hospitals don't let women do this, but treat birth as a medical crisis. If a woman is really listening to her body, however, and in tune with it, the rhythms come in waves – both the rhythms of contractions right through the first stage, and the bearing down urges in the second stage. Often there is a team of people standing over the mother and saying, 'Come on, mother, take a deep breath and *push*. Come on, *push* . . . *push* . . . *push*. . . . Come on, you can do better than that. . . . Hold your breath . . . and *push* . . . *push*. . . .' There she is with her eyes popping out of her head, little blood vessels breaking in her cheeks and eyes, straining and groaning. In fact it's an awful waste of energy, and she's not helping the baby get born. Moreover her prolonged breath-holding may well be cutting down the oxygen reaching the baby. She looks quite obviously in distress, which can reduce the amount of oxygenated blood flowing through the placenta to the baby. Recent studies by a very eminent obstetrician have shown that if a mother holds her breath for longer than six seconds there is a risk that she may cut down the oxygen reaching the baby, and yet people in hospitals still coax and cajole and command women to push.

My book *The Good Birth Guide*,* is a guide to hospitals that will listen to mothers and ask them how they would like to have their babies. In fact, the hospitals that have a totally sympathetic attitude to mothers. Although I haven't seen all these hospitals and don't know them at first hand, I believe we can learn a lot from women's experiences of them. Mothers have a great deal to contribute towards making things better for other women. When the book was first published I was very nervous about the response I might get from a lot of very angry doctors and midwives. Strangely enough, though, I had many letters of support and a good deal of follow-up, in that obstetricians, paediatricians and hospital administrators are now writing to me about changes in their hospitals, sometimes even sending a copy of their entry in *The Good Birth Guide*, numbering the criticisms and then telling me what they have done about them. In all the work I do I want to be a catalyst for change.

*Published by Fontana

SACKCLOTH AND ASHES

Patrick Galvin is an Irish poet and playwright

My father did not believe in women. He recognized the fact that they were there, he conceded their usefulness about the house, but he was not convinced of their intelligence. My mother, on the other hand, believed strongly in men. She knew that they were all raving mad, totally destructive, and an albatross around the neck of any woman who had the misfortune to marry one. But she was also religious – she believed in God, and she firmly believed that her place in this world was one of suffering and penance.

My mother worked. From the day and hour when she was able to stand on her own two feet she worked, and was made to work, for men. In her youth she looked after the needs of her brothers. When she married she looked after her husband, while he worked outside the house at what he considered to be work of national importance. What this work consisted of was never clearly defined, since for most of his life my father was officially unemployed.

During the bad old days, which for my mother meant living on a neighbour's charity and feeding her eight children on my father's meagre dole money, she managed to find extra work scrubbing other people's floors and taking in laundry. Her day began at 5.30 in the morning. She cooked my father's breakfast before she left the house, cooked his dinner when she returned in the evenings, and spent another few hours mending the family's clothes before finally retiring to bed. My father took all this for granted. It would never occur to him to make a meal or darn a sock. That, after all, was women's work.

On Sundays my father and mother went to church; they were true believers. In church the women sat on one side of the altar and the men sat on the other. The centre aisle was reserved for the upper classes. Here the sexes were permitted to mingle, presumably on the grounds that the upper classes were less sinful and less open to temptations of the flesh. My mother said nothing. My father might have said something, but he would not argue with the elders of his church. On Ash Wednesday my mother attended church an hour before she began her daily round of scrubbing and washing. Head lowered beneath her black shawl, she walked to the altar rail to receive the ashes. The priest smeared the ashes across her forehead, and the green ash fell on her blouse and stained her existence. She accepted her guilt. She accepted the Fall of Adam. And she accepted that she and her kind were responsible for the sufferings of mankind.

She was the woman. Her breasts proved it. Her smile proved it. Her gentle hands – raw from scrubbing floors – proved it beyond any shadow of a doubt. Not a day passed when she didn't have to work out her salvation. Not a night passed when she didn't have to rise from her bed, suckle her youngest child, and prepare breakfast for the older children who had to be made ready for school. When she left the house to begin her extra day's work she was already exhausted. And when she died her face bore the marks of crucified women the world over.

I did not attend her funeral. I stood at the chapel gate and watched the lid of her coffin being nailed down by men. I watched her coffin being carried to the graveyard on the shoulders of men. She would be lowered into the ground by men. She would be prayed over by a male priest, and she would be forgiven at last for all the sins she had never committed. In my darkest dreams she wears sackcloth and ashes. On a new dawn she rises above all men, a blazing resurrection.

CRISPY LEMON CAKE

Mary Berry's recipe is for a quick, one-stage cake with an unusual topping

4 oz (125 g) soft margarine
1 level teaspoon baking powder
6 oz (175 g) self-raising flour
6 oz (175 g) caster sugar
2 eggs
4 tablespoons milk
finely grated rind of 1 lemon

Icing
juice of 1 lemon
4 oz (125 g) caster sugar

Pre-heat the oven to 350°F (180°C, gas mark 4). Grease an 8 inch (20 cm) round cake tin and line it with greased greaseproof paper. Put the margarine, baking powder, flour, sugar, eggs and milk into a large bowl with the lemon rind and beat well for about 2 minutes. Turn into the cake tin and bake for 50 to 60 minutes, or until the cake has shrunk from the sides of the tin and springs back when pressed with a finger in the centre.

While the cake is baking, put the lemon juice and sugar in a bowl or cup and stir until blended. When the sponge comes out of the oven, spread the lemon paste over the top while still hot. Leave in the tin until quite cold, then turn out, remove the paper and store in an airtight tin.

NEW YORK ON PARADE

Helene Hanff

I wish to enlist your sympathy for the poor millionaires who live on Fifth Avenue, in New York's most expensive town houses and co-op apartments. With the coming of the warm months, they're braced for a long succession of ethnic parades up Fifth Avenue, Sunday after Sunday. Pulaski Day and Von Steuben Day parades are held in honour of European generals who fought in the American War of Independence. Pulaski was a Pole, von Steuben was a German – so the Pulaski Day parade is organized by Polish New Yorkers, the Von Steuben Day parade by German New Yorkers. For other ethnic groups there are parades on Greek Independence Day, Puerto Rico Day, Salute to Israel Day, Philippine Independence Day, and so forth, including Captive Nations Day for Armenian, Bulgarian, Czech, Hungarian, Lithuanian and Romanian New Yorkers.

All these parades go straight up Fifth Avenue, which means that at 8 a.m. of a spring Sunday the occupants of a town house are wakened by the boom-boom of the drum and the raucous blare of a trumpet, as the first marching band tunes up under their windows. It will be followed by twenty more marching bands, and the millionaires will get no peace for the rest of the day. They formed community action groups and demanded that the city issue parade permits only on weekdays. But this was fought by Fifth Avenue merchants, since parade crowds impede shoppers and are bad for business. So the millionaires demanded that the city move its Sunday parades to some other avenue. This the city authorities

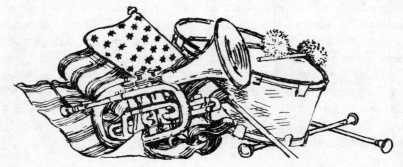

could not do – you can't give one ethnic group the right to march up Fifth Avenue, and tell all the other groups to march some-where else, and a century ago, the first New York ethnic group to hold a parade had its right to use Fifth Avenue written into the City Charter. That group still holds the city's biggest and most popular parade, popular even with the millionaires since it's never on a Sunday. The parade is held on 17 March, and when that falls on a Sunday it's held on the eighteenth, because the parade is in honour of St Patrick's Day, and there's a reviewing stand in front of St Patrick's Cathedral.

St Patrick's Day is unique in New York. For reasons known to nobody, on 17 March the entire city becomes Irish. Everybody wears a green tie or blouse to work; florists do a booming business in green buttonhole carnations; bakeries and supermarkets feature cakes with green icing and shamrock-shaped cookies; and ice cream parlours do a great trade in mint and pistachio ice cream. But there was one never-to-be-forgotten St Patrick's Day, back in the sixties, that surpassed them all.

New York has always had a large Irish Catholic population and a small Irish Protestant population. One year in the sixties the Mayor of Dublin, Robert Briscoe, was to be guest of honour at the St Patrick's Day parade. The newspapers announced that Robert Briscoe was not an Irish Catholic, nor yet an Irish Protestant, but – Heaven bless us – an Irish Jew. The Jewish population of New York went completely out of its mind. Cohen's clothing store and Goldberg's meat market painted green O-apostrophes on their signs and became O'Cohen's and O'Goldberg's for the day. Deli-catessens sold green bagels, and kosher restaurants served green matzo balls and green noodles in their soup. Whole Hebrew schools turned out for the parade as the annual sea of green floats, marching bands and schoolgirls in green shorts rolled past the Cathedral, before the three dignitaries on the reviewing stand: Jewish Mayor Briscoe of Dublin, Protestant Mayor Lindsay of New York, and the Catholic Archbishop between them.

SUMMER

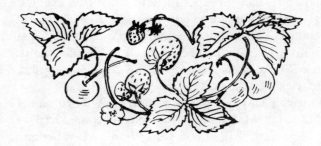

COUNTRY DIARY

Robin Page on the countryside in August

These days the whole pace of the harvest has changed. In the old days of the binder it was more restful and relaxed and the corn could be cut when it was damp. Now, with combine harvesters, you have to wait until the grain is really dry, because if it's cut damp it heats up and goes mouldy in the bins. So nowadays there's one great frenetic rush – as soon as things are dry the farmers are going all the hours that God gives. It's hard work: you get covered from head to foot with dust and dirt and end up grimier than a coal miner. The romance has gone out of harvesting – though it's still pleasant, because you get a great deal of satisfaction watching the amount of standing corn steadily being reduced.

At the end of the day, when you walk home feeling tired, one of the things you notice is the silence, because the birds have stopped singing at this time of the year. The problems of territory and love have gone, and it's relaxing to walk home at dusk in that silence.

Another thing we notice during the harvest is whether the pheasants have done well, because as the corn is cut the families of young birds fly. It's part of the countryman's strange attitude towards pheasants that throughout the summer he's looking for them and protecting them, and as they fly from the corn he feels very satisfied and pleased that they've done quite well despite the wet; then, as soon as the shooting season comes, it's different,

76

because he likes roast pheasant. It's very contradictory, really.

As the corn goes you also see stoats and weasels from time to time, and small predators, and the odd fox will come out. I found something completely new to me recently, in an unusual fox dropping. I don't make a habit of studying fox droppings, but this one caught my eye because it was full of fresh garden peas. It shows how adaptable foxes are and how varied their diet is, because they will eat pheasants and chickens but they will also scavenge anything – garden peas, beetles, worms. This adaptability is part of the fascination of foxes.

Harvest flowers were also to be seen: field scabious – which no doubt most people see – knapweed, round-leaved fluellen, and scarlet pimpernel. The last of these is one of my favourites: it's known as the poor man's weather glass, because when it's open the weather's good, and when it closes it's going to rain.

There are a lot of young ducks on our village pond – eleven plus the parents – and they have become part of the village family. As the pensioners go by the pond to get their pensions they throw

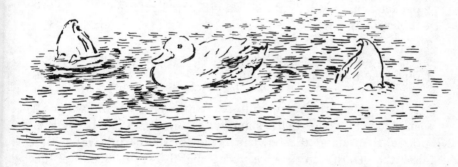

them bits of bread. There was great alarm during a recent August when they suddenly disappeared, and people said the gipsies had poached them, and that they were going to be roasted. Somebody even suggested that paraffin had been poured on the pond to frighten them off. In fact all they had done was learn to fly, and having discovered their freedom they had made off. One evening I saw them come crashing down out of the sky on to the pond, and everybody was happy again.

On the farm we had guinea fowl which also started flying. They are lovely little birds. We've got Muscovy ducks, too, but they didn't hatch any fertile eggs this year, partly because for most of the summer the old drake thought he was a goose, and spent his time chasing the geese instead of going with his duck, which was very unfortunate for everybody. We also had two beautiful calves recently. I get a lot of pleasure out of watching a successful calving; the small animal comes out hot and steaming, the mother lows and licks it, and then it looks around with amazement. We still have the 'bisnings', which is the thick milk produced just after a cow has calved. It's got a lot of antibodies in it for the calf. We heat it up, add sugar, put it in the oven and eat it like an egg custard: it's delicious.

RASPBERRY MOUSSE

Mary Berry's recipe serves six people

¼ pint (150 ml) fruit purée – raspberry or strawberry
juice of ½ lemon
1 packet or 1 rounded tablespoon powdered gelatine
3 tablespoons water
3 eggs
3 to 4 oz (90 to 125 g) caster sugar, or to taste
¼ pint (150 ml) whipping cream

Mix the purée with the lemon juice. Put the gelatine and water in a small bowl or cup. Let it stand for 3 minutes until it becomes a sponge, then stand the bowl in a pan of simmering water and allow the gelatine to dissolve. Keep slightly warm. Separate the eggs and put the yolks, fruit purée and sugar in a bowl. Stand it over a pan of simmering water and whisk until thick and creamy, which will take about 10 minutes. Remove from the heat and continue whisking until cool, then pour in the gelatine, whisking all the time until well blended. Whisk the egg whites with an electric or hand rotary whisk until fairly stiff. Whip the cream. Fold first the cream and then the egg whites into the fruit mixture until smoothly blended. Pour into a 2½ pint (1.5 l) dish, smooth the top and leave in a cool place to set.

JOURNEY TO AMRITSAR

Judy King is the pseudonym of a former army nurse who served in India during the Second World War. The story was read as a serial on Woman's Hour

In May 1945 I was working as an army nursing sister in a British military hospital in Poona – specifically on the officers' ward of the tuberculosis block. The majority of patients were white, but the ward had several side wards reserved for Indian officers. No conflict arose between white and Indian patients, though there was a tacit avoidance of each other. The main problem, apart from the lowering nature of tuberculosis, which affects the patient morally, physically and spiritually, was nostalgia. It was most marked among the white patients, whose longing for home after years of bitter jungle fighting became almost pathological.

With the Indian patients the problem was different – they were already on home ground, and their attitude towards TB was more fatalistic. What they most deeply resented was the enforced regimentation of their idleness. The worst were the Sikhs, and of the Sikhs Flight-Lieutenant Singh Maan was the villain of the piece. He was a gravely sick man with infiltration in both lungs, but he brought all sorts of troubles down on his own head by virtue of his defiance. Physical infirmity is intolerable to a martial Sikh anyway, and he made no secret of the fact that he resented his disease, British Army discipline, and above all his enforced subjection to the care of women – white, foreign women at that! Yet in my association with this man, brief though it was, I learned more about India than in the whole of the rest of my time there.

Though by heredity a martial Sikh, Singh Maan had been a farmer in civilian life, and his home was far away in the north. When I first joined the ward I knew no more about him than that, but one brief glimpse at his notes was enough to tell me he would never farm again. He was confined to bed not so much by doctor's orders, which he consistently ignored anyway, as by the gravity of his condition. He was always clamouring to be sent home, and many efforts had been made by the hospital administration to achieve this. However, the demands of a sick Sikh officer were unlikely to receive priority attention with a full-scale war still raging against the Japanese. Delay was inevitable, and by the time

79

a passage by air to Delhi seemed a distinct probability, the state of his lungs was such that medical opinion was unanimous against the advisability of flying.

So it came about that arrangements were made to transport him to his home by train under medical escort. He was asked if there were any particular members of the ward staff whom he would like to accompany him, and he chose myself and a somewhat bizarre ward orderly named Hill. Hill was tall, physically powerful, and full of the quick, caustic wit of the Londoner born and bred. He had been down-graded from a combatant unit due to an eye injury sustained in Burma, and had taken the whole process as a personal insult to his valour. He dressed himself in a weird assembly of clothes, mostly, I imagine, to offset the military 'disgrace' of being attached to the 'meat waggons' – a disrespectful term he used to describe all medical units. When off duty he wore a filthy, battered and much prized bush hat cocked at a defiant angle. Regulations demanded that he wore the usual bush shirt and shorts, but what shorts! They must have been the shortest shorts ever, and to make his appearance even odder he insisted on wearing – whenever he thought he could get away with it – a pair of mosquito boots of the type used in jungle warfare. Whether all this helped to create for him the illusion of being back in the jungle no one ever found out, but whatever the strangeness of his garb, or the reluctance of his presence with us, he was nevertheless a very good orderly. For this reason alone he was never put on a charge for being improperly dressed. This, then, was the orderly who would be accompanying us, together with another, not from our ward, by the name of Morgan.

Matron told me I was to prepare for a long train journey on the Frontier Mail to Amritsar. I was to take all the equipment I needed from the hospital stores, and collect warrants and a movement order from the registrar. I was somewhat shaken when she announced that Amritsar was some 1,500 miles from Bombay, and that the journey would take two nights and two days.

'What if he dies on the train?' I asked.

'Stop the train and inform the guard', she replied without hesitation. 'They won't carry dead bodies on Indian trains, so you will have to arrange to have it put off at the nearest military post, and they must take charge of it.'

The next question hit me like a bomb. 'How do I stop the

Frontier Mail?' On Indian trains I had never seen anything remotely like a communication cord, and there were no corridors.

Matron herself was a bit foxed by this one, so she rapidly switched from negative to positive. 'Sister! All this talk about dead bodies and stopping express trains. It's a live patient you are taking, and your job is to get him there alive! Stop fussing – if you have to stop the train you'll stop it all right. Now listen to me. . . .'

She told me the story behind Singh Maan's fanatical desire to get home. Apparently he had fifteen-month-old twin sons whom he had never seen. He also had large holdings of agricultural land in the Punjab, the rights to which had to be put into the hands of these babies before he died. There was family conflict about this, inasmuch as his younger brother was losing no time in his efforts to filch the legal land rights from the legitimate heirs. Lawyers in the Punjab were powerless, since according to Sikh law the transfer of land had to be made in the physical presence of the contracting parties.

'There is one thing we have promised him,' Matron said, 'and that is the dignity of a full-dress escort when he arrives in his home town. Orientals are very particular in matters concerned with "face", so you will please make sure to wear a clean white uniform dress and veil as the train pulls in to Amritsar. And you will need your bearer with you. Send him to the registrar for his fare – he must travel third class. Good luck, Sister! This is a bit tough, I know, but you'll do it.'

'Phew!' I thought as I went in search of solace and advice in the mess. 'What an assignment.' Several of the older sisters regarded me with a mixture of amusement and scorn when I gave the broad outline of my mission.

'All dangerously ills are supposed to travel with a medical officer – that much, I'm sure, is in King's Regulations', said one.

'So that makes you a right green one, doesn't it?' said another. 'Never, never, *never* volunteer.'

'But I didn't', I protested.

'Oh, you're a volunteer all right. They couldn't possibly order you on a trip like that.'

I must have looked somewhat crestfallen, for they all burst out laughing, and I got quite angry.

'I'm going at the patient's request', I said sharply, with all the dignity I could muster.

They had no answer for that one, but as I swept haughtily out of the door someone murmured: 'You'll never get him there alive.'

I knew there was some truth in this. It bothered me all night.

I spent the next day trailing around the hospital compound in boiling sun collecting equipment for the journey. My first call was to the quartermaster's store. Jovial and helpful at first, the guardian angel of 'spoons, tea' and 'plates, dinner' soon became suspicious and hostile as the list of my requirements grew longer and longer.

'Who said you could take all this?' he growled. 'You'll have to sign for everything in triplicate. . . . Anyway where the heck is Amritsar?' he asked finally.

I told him.

His face grew long with what I took for fatherly concern. 'They didn't ought to be sending a young sister like you all that way on your own', he observed, sorting the utensils into piles. Then he added, 'Not with all my stuff, they didn't', which rather spoiled the effect.

I deposited the swag in my room and proceeded to medical stores. '*Morphia*', echoed the sergeant behind the counter, as though it were an extremely rare species of vermin. 'And what for? . . . Who said so? . . . Where's your authority?' were fired at me in quick succession.

I stated my case firmly, being careful to drop the name of Matron every other word.

The sergeant was unimpressed. 'Can't get morphia on the mere say-so of a matron', he said.

In the end it was the colonel himself who had to smooth the way, as morphia came under the direct supervision of the deputy area commander.

I was now officially 'off the strength' for the purpose of the trip, so I decided to call the team together. We sat on the verandah of a disused ward. Private Hill had for once dressed himself more conventionally, and was full of bright suggestions. After the obstructive morning I'd had I was only too glad to have his cheery comments, and indeed this strong and sensible cockney was to prove a pillar of strength. Private Morgan, on the other hand, was obviously not going to be the brightest of helpmates. A sad little man of thirty-five or more, he had been called up late in the war and had been in India only five weeks. But even Morgan was to

82

rally bravely in the moments of crisis which lay ahead of us. Chota Lal, my little Indian bearer, squatting on the floor beside me, was as excited as a child at Christmas, though he made little secret of the fact that he thought we were all quite mad. He chirped and twittered until in irritation I sent him off to get cups of tea for us from the mess while we began to study the movement order. Couched in typical army language, this document informed us tersely that various stations and places had been signalled to expect and provide for us.

'Bah!' said Hill with disdain. 'If you ask me that's not worth the paper it's written on.' His observation was to prove only too true. . . .

As the bright rose tints of the morning filled my room I realized this was it. This was *the day*!

Chota Lal came in with tea and biscuits. He was full of excitement. 'Quick, quick, missy-sahib, morning time come. You get up. Today we go to Punjab.' He plonked the tea down, spilling most of it into the saucer.

His sense of urgency infected me and I got up, although it was only 6.30 a.m. There was a special early breakfast for me in the mess. I then went to the ward, where I'd asked both orderlies to meet me. They were sitting on the steps with all the baggage, and together we went up to the ward. The day staff had not yet come on and the night sister was in charge.

In the Indian side wards there was a sense of expectancy. All eyes watched me as I approached the patient with Night Sister. Singh Maan lay quiet in his bed. His hair had been immaculately dressed, I imagined by one of the other Sikh officers. 'How on earth am I going to keep it like that?' I thought as I looked at him.

'Good morning, Singh Maan', I said. 'Are you ready for your long journey home?'

He said that he was, then added with unexpected courtesy, 'It is good of you to come so far with me, Sister.'

Night Sister and I moved away from the bed as the other Sikhs came forward to say goodbye. One man after another approached and bowed low, hands pressed palm to palm in the formal gesture of salutation. When they had finished no one spoke. The two orderlies waiting in the doorway approached with the stretcher, and gently we lifted the dying Sikh on to it. Our journey had begun.

The big army ambulance was waiting by the ward steps. As we were finishing the loading I was approached by a corporal from the registrar's office, who saluted me smartly and handed over an official-looking envelope marked 'Urgent'. I glanced quickly at it, then stuffed it into the pocket of my bush jacket and climbed into the ambulance. The ride into Poona took only minutes, and getting on to the train for Bombay was simple enough. The Deccan Queen was an express, stopping once only, and did the 120-odd-mile run to Bombay in just under three hours. We had a double first-class compartment to ourselves, and the morning was still cool. After settling the patient comfortably I remembered the envelope and pulled it from my pocket. On opening it I found it was a signed authority from the colonel, to be used on the Frontier Mail in the event of the patient's death. So Matron had taken that one seriously after all. Hill watched me inquisitively. I put the message back in my pocket and deliberately turned my attention to the scenery outside.

At times the railway climbed to a height of nearly three thousand feet above sea-level. The countryside was rocky and barren, villages were scanty, and the heat gradually increased. We gave the patient a drink twice; he didn't complain, and spoke very little. Morgan complained, however, about his feet, and Hill gave him a lecture on the folly of wearing new shoes on a 'joy-ride like this', as he put it.

As we plunged down towards the coastal plain, the heat turned from dry to moist, and by noon the atmosphere was very unpleasant indeed. Every effort caused violent perspiration, and at Victoria Terminus the operation of getting Singh Maan out of the train on to the stretcher and to a shaded part of the platform was exhausting. I left him in the charge of the orderlies while I went to the railway transport office to see about transport to Central Station. The officer had gone to lunch, so I had to deal with a corporal left in charge of the office. I presented the movement order confidently and was met with blank surprise.

'We've had no signal', said the corporal.

Fine start, I thought. 'You *must* have', I insisted. He eyed me doubtfully, then said, 'Just a minute, Sister.' He went inside and I could hear him on the telephone. There was some argument, and

84

then he hung up and reappeared. 'We've had nothing from the hospital at Poona', he said, as though this were the final word.

'I can't help that. I've got a very sick patient out on your dirty platform. We've got to get him over to Central Station and we are not going to carry him there!'

'Well, what can I do?' complained the corporal. 'We've got no transport for you – how about the IWA?'

I pushed my cap on the back of my head and wiped my perspiring brow while gaining breath to yell at him. 'The Indian Women's Aid Society! We are supposed to be *military*.'

The corporal shut his eyes while the storm raged, then he said, 'Yes, I know. But they've got some jolly good ambulances. Shall I give them a ring?'

I had to give in. I sank in a perspiring heap on to a chair, where I waited for the best part of ten minutes while the corporal shifted the army's load of responsibility on to the IWA. How undignified, I thought. Less than two hundred miles from Poona and here we are, already enlisting the help of a voluntary body. I felt depressed.

Hill came along to find out the cause of the hold-up.

'Told you so', he said smugly. 'In this perishing army once one place has got shot of you you're on your tod. I can tell you – I've had some!'

'Oh, shut up', I snapped, surprising Hill with my sharp and unladylike manner.

IWA headquarters were, however, helpful, and eventually a luxurious ambulance arrived. We wasted no time in getting Singh Maan out of the station, where the dust had brought on a fit of coughing which left him grey-faced and spent. Once inside the ambulance I had to attend to him. He was too exhausted to speak, but was quite conscious, and with repeated applications of iced water to his face and neck he began to revive a little. It was a journey of several miles right across the teeming, boiling heart of Bombay, and by the time we arrived at the big Victorian pile known as Central Station Singh Maan had lapsed into a comfortable doze. He protested feebly at being moved again, but the first-class waiting-room was spacious and airy, with a plentiful supply of large electric fans in the ceiling, and fortunately devoid of other travellers.

Our next priority was food. It wasn't difficult to get lightly poached eggs and bread and butter from the first-class restaurant, and I slowly fed Singh Maan with this. I sent Chota Lal to the bazaar for mangoes and other fruit for the journey, and to get his own food. The orderlies too had gone for a meal, and so for a time I was alone with the patient. The effort of eating and drinking was obviously great. He closed his eyes and I thought he had fallen asleep, but after a moment he opened them and said:

'Am I going to get home, Sister?'

'Yes', I replied without hesitation, and seeing him smile added: 'I have promised the gods.'

There was a pause. 'Only one God for the Sikhs', he whispered.

I wanted to ask him more but, fearing the added strain this would put upon him, I said instead, 'Will you let my try to do your hair for you?'

He had never allowed any of the sisters to touch his hair in Poona, but to my surprise he said 'Yes.'

My first attempt was amateurish and clumsy. I was afraid to loosen the bun too much in case I couldn't get it back together again, so I combed the hair upwards and away from the face as best I could. When my fidgety fumblings began to distress him I gave up.

The orderlies came back looking fresher and cleaner. Preparing to depart myself, I asked Hill to go to the railway transport office in my absence to make inquiries about our passage on the Frontier Mail, which was due to leave at six o'clock that evening.

I had a bath and a meal and when I returned nearly two hours later Singh Maan was asleep. So was Chota Lal, outside the door. Only Morgan remained on guard. There was no sign of Hill and the fact that he'd been gone so long seemed to spell trouble, so I set out immediately to find him.

Bombay Central Station is vast, and I had some difficulty finding the transport offices. When I did it took several minutes to locate Hill.

'It's just no cop, Sister', he said shortly. 'As far as I can make out they haven't even booked us on the perishing train!'

'Oh, rubbish', I said, trying to sound calm. 'Who have you seen?'

'About everybody except the commanding officer', he replied wearily. 'The sarge in there's trying to contact the CO now.'

'Well, let's get in there, then. We can't hang about here all day.'

I paused. 'No. You go back upstairs with Morgan – this is going to take everything I've got, and I'd rather do it alone.'

The CO was a regular major, and a very harassed man. 'Sister, I can't get you on to the Frontier Mail with only two days' notice – it can't be done!' He waved the movement order at me.

'Two days!' I repeated. 'But I was ordered on this job more than a week ago. I thought all arrangements had been made.'

'Two days', he said again. 'Now, the question is – what am I going to do with you?'

'I can save you the trouble of working that one out, Major', I announced coolly. 'You are going to get us to Amritsar.'

He frowned. 'And just how am I supposed to do that? Do you realize the weight of military traffic I am having to handle here? Whole regiments on the move. Wounded and sick being evacuated out of Burma. Half the world's here in Bombay, and you expect me to halt everything to get you and some Sikh up to Amritsar?'

I began to protest, but he shut me up.

'Oh yes, I know about this. I've been in contact with your registrar at Poona on more than one occasion about this man, and I told them six weeks ago that the chance of air-conditioned accommodation on the Frontier Mail was out of the question. It's reserved months in advance by Delhi High Command for senior officers, by leaders of the Congress Party, by Indian bankers, rajahs and I don't know who else.' He waved the movement order at me. 'They should never have sent you out of Poona. You will just have to take this patient back.'

These final words aroused all my obstinacy and determination. 'I'm not taking him back', I said. 'The man is dying and he has the right to die in his own home.'

I spent the next five minutes telling the major Singh Maan's story. At the end of it he leaned back in his chair.

'How old are you, Sister?' he asked sharply.

'Twenty-four', I replied promptly.

'How long in the army?'

This time my answer wasn't so prompt. 'Six months – but I know what war's about. I did my training in London right through the Blitz. I'm no baby.'

This brought a roar of laughter, and I knew I had won. The major pressed a buzzer on his desk and in came a sergeant, saluting smartly.

'Briggs! Get me a copy of the passenger list for the Frontier Mail going out tonight.'

'Sir', barked the sergeant and disappeared.

'Now, Sister, I will tell you what I propose to do.' He would cancel the bookings of any junior officers going up to Kashmir on leave – there were bound to be some, he said. He would requisition their coupé, which would be four-berthed and large enough to take the patient, myself, and the two orderlies travelling together. The bearer would be accommodated in the third-class servants' carriage at the back of the first-class coaches. The dining-coach was separate and couldn't be reached except at scheduled stops provided for this purpose. Indian food would be available, but would have to be fetched and carried for the patient. I said I had made provision for this, and he expressed satisfaction. The sergeant then returned with the list, and the major studied it.

'Good. Better than I thought', he said. 'Three second lieutenants travelling together, plus an Ambala professor. Right – they've had it! Sergeant! Cancel these bookings.' He indicated the names with a pencil. 'Send out a call for the military – they must be around by now – and tell all three to report here. Tell the station-master that the Ambala professor must be contacted over their tannoy. He'll have to be transferred to the Delhi Express. No arguments. Military priority. We'll give him a chit later if he insists.'

He got up and paced the floor. 'Now, that's got you on the train. Where was I? Ah yes, ice', he said.

I looked puzzled.

'Have you travelled at all on Indian trains?'

When I said I hadn't much, he explained the procedure for keeping cool. I would have to buy blocks of ice to place in the lead tray provided in the compartment. There were icing stations all along the route, he said. A note of anxiety came into his voice. 'No experience of the London Blitz will prepare you for the sort of heat and discomfort you are going to hit a thousand miles out from here in the plains, Sister. Do you think your patient will stand it?'

'I don't know', I admitted. 'The matron said I was to stop the train if he dies.'

'Hell's bells!' exploded the major. 'You can't stop this train!'

Rather timidly I said I had expressed the same fear to the matron.

'Huh!' he snorted. 'What other tom-fool tales did they tell you back in Poona? Do you realize that this train is the best part of a quarter of a mile long? It's no local excursion puff-puff! . . . Now back to ice – you'll need one block here, another at Ratlam, one at Kotah and the last one possibly at Delhi. Twelve rupees is the standard price – don't let them overcharge you. . . . Oh, and you can have this splendid bit of fiction back.' He thrust the movement order at me.

I didn't move, and he sat down in exasperation.

'Well! What now?' he said.

I felt frightened and on the verge of tears, and though I would have died rather than show it, he knew, and his tone softened.

'I know, I know – you've got no money.' He shook his head. 'Right. Next on the agenda – field cashier and signals office. Can't have young sisters trailing all round India with no money and lacking proper authority, can we?' I didn't know what to say and he went on, 'The army's all right when you get used to it. It has a tremendous aptitude for correcting its own mistakes as it goes along. You won't be alone, Sister. We are in touch with the stations right up to the frontier. You'll see.'

I felt tremendously relieved. In a flood of gratitude I tried to thank him, but he cut me short.

'All in a day's work, ma'am. Now I'm going to put you in charge of Briggs to get your money and send your signal. But take my word for it, they won't turn you back now.' He buzzed for the sergeant, said he would see me again when aboard the train, and the interview was over.

Outside the office another problem occurred to me. What about Singh Maan? I had to break the news to him that he was about to face one of the toughest journeys of his life. I knew what his answer would be – to go on, no matter what. But I felt I must at least tell him, so I asked the sergeant to wait for me while I did so.

Back in the waiting-room Singh Maan was awake and restless. Hill was bathing his face and Morgan was peeling a mango. Even Chota Lal, still outside the door, looked solemn and alarmed. Hill spoke to me on one side.

'I'm glad you're back', he said shortly. 'He's been fussing like the devil, and his pulse has shot up.'

'Never mind – everything's settled.' I went over to Singh Maan. 'Sister, you've been so long', he said. 'There is trouble?'

I didn't beat about the bush. 'Yes, we can't get an air-conditioned coupé.'

To my surprise he took this quite calmly.

I told him what had happened, and what a strain the journey would put upon him, ending up with: 'Well, there it is. Do you think you can make it, or would you rather we took you back to Poona?'

He closed his eyes for a moment, then opened them again. 'You know the answer', he whispered.

I felt his pulse. It was, as Hill had said, very rapid. 'You must rest', I said. 'It is 3.30 now. The train doesn't leave until six. I'll give you something to make you sleep.'

He protested, but a fit of coughing stopped him short, and I had to support his shoulders until it subsided. The gauze which I took away from his mouth was tinged with blood. I took the morphia out of the kit-bag. He didn't move as I put the needle into his arm.

'Watch him carefully', I said to Hill. 'I don't want a haemorrhage now. I'm going to get some money and send a signal back to Poona for authority for us to go on. I shall be in the field cashier's office or the signals room – wherever that is – if you want me.'

Outside the waiting-room Sergeant Briggs met me with a grin. 'How did you do it, Sister?' he asked, and for the moment I couldn't think what he was talking about. He went on: 'I've been with him over a year and I've never known the old man turn a train out for anybody before – it must be your bonny brown eyes.'

I tried to look dignified. 'He did it for a dying Sikh officer,' I said, 'not for me.'

On the Frontier Mail

The transaction with the field cashier took very little time and I came away 100 rupees the richer. I marvelled at how easy it was to get money in the army when you knew how.

The excursion to the signals room took longer. All the lines were booked, and the place was a hive of activity. Briggs, however, knew his way about and eventually commandeered a line.

'There you are, Sister', he said. 'All yours!'

The corporal operator looked up at me expectantly.

'Gosh!' I said. 'I don't know how to put this in army language.'

90

'Don't try', said Briggs. 'They'll never understand it at the other end if you do', and we all laughed. Between the three of us, however, we did make up a fairly impressive-sounding signal, which ran something like this: FROM SISTER I/C SICK PARTY AMRITSAR TO 126 IBGH POONA ATTENTION COMMANDING OFFICER TOP PRIORITY STOP NO AIR CONDITIONED ACCOMMODATION FRONTIER MAIL STOP FIRST CLASS COACH WHOLE PARTY TOGETHER OFFERED STOP REQUEST AUTHORITY PROCEED OR RETURN POONA STOP.

I thanked Briggs for his help and he said he would be up later to see how we were getting on. 'The reply to your signal should be through in a couple of hours', he added, and I began to feel like a veteran.

'If it's not, I'll go without it', I said.

He gave me a broad, chummy grin. As the major had said, we were not alone any more.

The atmosphere when I returned to the waiting-room was one of peace and calm. Chota Lal was asleep outside the door, and Singh Maan had apparently not moved since I left him. I felt his pulse and it had steadied somewhat. He opened his eyes and smiled. The morphia had had a blessed effect.

'No more coughing?' I asked Hill.

'Nope', he replied. 'How'd you get on, Sister? Everything fixed?'

I assured him that it was, and that we were merely awaiting the reply to the signal. Before he could make his usual gloomy comment I forestalled him. 'Yes . . . I-know-what-it-will-be', I said. 'I've found out quite a bit about the army this afternoon, and quite a lot of what you say is right. Most times it's a bloody shambles.'

Hill's eyebrows shot up in surprise.

'But it's not as bad as you make out by half, and surprisingly enough we will get to Amritsar, I think.'

'Cor blimey! We 'ave grown up, 'aven't we?' said Hill.

'And that's enough of your cheek!' I said without rancour.

He grinned, rubbed both hands together and said, 'Tea! What d'you say to me going foraging for a nice tray of char, Sister, eh?'

'Good idea', I said. . . .

At 5.30 p.m. Briggs arrived as he had promised. He said no reply had yet been received to my signal, and what did I propose to do?

'We'll go without it', I said.

'I thought perhaps you would', said Briggs. 'The old man said to give you a hand.'

We gathered our baggage together as silently as we could, in order to leave Singh Maan asleep until the last possible moment. The orderlies then took everything down to the train and Sergeant Briggs led the way. I stayed beside Singh Maan and everything was quiet.

Chota Lal peeped in shyly – being of low caste he hadn't the temerity to come inside. I beckoned to him. He still hesitated, and I had to hiss: 'Come in.' I motioned to him to sit beside me and he squatted on the floor clutching his bundle of belongings.

'We are going to need all your help', I whispered, and I told him of the arrangements that had been made.

He was delighted, as much by the excitement of the journey as by being made supernumerary personnel to a pukka military escort party.

'Now you go down and find your quarters and get settled into the train', I told him.

I sat on alone for several minutes, musing on the prospect before us. Would Singh Maan reach his home alive? The odds were set against him now. His small reserves of strength were being drained away slowly by each bout of coughing and restless anxiety.

The orderlies returned and with amazing gentleness laid the Sikh on to the stretcher. Singh Maan was hardly roused, but as he brushed past me he caught my hand. The strength of the grip was astonishing.

'All set', I murmured. 'Here we go.'

Half the population of Bombay seemed intent on boarding the train, but with the worthy Briggs to clear the way we got the stretcher through. The coupé was clean and roomy. It had its own bathroom and toilet, but unlike British trains there was no corridor. The bunks, four of them, were let in against the sides of the train – the bottom two fixed, the top pair hinged so that they could be pushed up out of the way when not in use. There was one upholstered armchair with wooden arms and legs. In the roof of the compartment were two fans, and underneath, as the major had said, a battered lead tray about three feet square and two feet deep, as yet empty of ice.

We got Singh Maan into the train, and then came the business of having the ice loaded. As with everything in the East, it had to be done with a good deal of noisy arguing and shouting, but Hill and Briggs between them cut this to a minimum. At ten minutes to six the major from the transport office came along the platform towards us. He had with him the guard of the train, an Anglo-Indian gentleman in immaculate white, complete with topee.

'I've told the guard all about you, Sister', said the major. 'If you – er – run into any difficulties, he will be able to help you.'

I knew that 'difficulties' meant the death of the patient.

Our departure was now imminent. The faint roar of steam could be heard above the babble of the crowds on the platform.

'Oh, Sister, I nearly forgot to give you this', the major said as he jumped out.

It was the reply signal from Poona, which I had forgotten all about. A quick glance told me our onward passage was confirmed. Then very slowly, amid a shrill chorus of whistles, the monstrous bulk of the Frontier Mail began to move.

It took us about half an hour to get ourselves ship-shape. While Hill and I did the chores, Morgan came into his own. He washed and tended the sick man with a gentleness which was astonishing, and finally shamed us all by braiding the tangled black hair and beard with confident efficiency. Singh Maan's face bore a look of battered exhaustion, but Morgan's clever management of his hair had at least given him once more the full dignity of a Sikh.

'Morgan has done your hair beautifully', I remarked.

He nodded faintly.

'How did you manage that?' I asked Morgan, remembering my own amateurish attempts.

'I'm a barber in civvy street', he replied.

For the first time he began to register as a person. 'Where is your home?' I asked him.

'Coventry', he replied, and said no more.

'That was very badly hit.'

'Yes . . . my wife and boy were killed', he said blankly.

Hill and I made no comment. What was there to say?

The great train headed north into the sunset and I stayed at the window to watch the ending of this day of frustration and anxiety. The Indian sunset never failed to impress me. It doesn't just 'get dark' in India – there is no twilight. As it descends towards the horizon, the sun seems to explode in a primitive protest against the eclipsing approach of night. For the brief space of ten minutes, certainly no more, the sky is orange, red and gold – then all the world is dark. I turned back into the compartment. Singh Maan was asleep.

At eight o'clock the train stopped at a small station, where the guard patrolled the platform shouting that there would be a ten-minute wait for passengers to enter the dining-car. Chota Lal's grinning face popped up at the window.

'You want me to get *khana*, Sister-sahib?' he asked.

'Yes', I said. 'Bring me light stuff, please – eggs, cold ham if they've got it, chutney, and hot milk in the flask.' I snatched up the small flask set aside for the patient, as well as two small china bowls which I thrust into his arms. 'And fish or chicken curry and rice in those.'

'No ham, missy!' he announced. 'Muslim cook in charge of kitchens!'

'Oh, you know what to get', I yelled crossly, and pushed him out of the door.

'Chitty! Chitty!' he screeched.

Oh, those infernal chits! I rummaged in my hold-all for paper and pencil. Then Chota Lal hurried off into the dark, followed by the two orderlies.

Singh Maan was still asleep, and I gazed out into the night. There was no moon, and this increased the density of blackness around the shining stars. My three musketeers came back with the food not a moment too soon. Before we had time to organize things the train was on the move again. It was too late for Chota Lal to return to the servants' compartment, so after setting out the food for us he retired to a corner by the door. With the renewed jolting of the train Singh Maan woke up. He started up with a cry and obviously didn't realize where he was, but a few words from us reassured him.

'Have a little of this food', I coaxed. 'It looks and smells very good.' I held out the two bowls for his inspection, but he showed little interest and asked what the time was.

'I thought I had slept all night', he sighed. 'Still so far away . . . so far away.'

I tried again with the food, and he agreed to have some warm milk. It did the trick, and he took a fair portion of the curried chicken with rice. This was good going and would give him some

94

added strength, but he soon began to use this up by talking. His eyes were too bright, and although I didn't bother to take his temperature I knew it must be up. I tried to quieten him down. I washed his face and neck with cold water, but still he insisted on chatting about the Punjab and his twin sons. Sometimes the words were incoherent, sometimes in Punjabi. I grew alarmed. His pulse was rising, and after half an hour I whispered to Hill, 'Get the morphia out.'

Singh Maan barely noticed the needle entering his arm, but he coughed suddenly, and with increasing anxiety I wiped away the specks of bright red blood on his lips.

'Oh no!' I murmured. 'Not that – now now!' I looked up into Hill's face as he bent forward handing me the swabs. We both knew that a major haemorrhage from the lungs would finish him, here and now. And what could we do?

But the morphia did its work quickly and well, and Singh Maan slipped away into drugged sleep. For nearly an hour we watched him, applying iced gauze swabs to his forehead and neck all the time. Occasionally he coughed feebly, but there was no further sign of the haemorrhage we had feared. The heat was still intense. Both Morgan and Chota Lal were asleep.

'Let's turn in', I said to Hill. 'Wake Morgan up. He can watch for a few hours.'

I went into the toilet annexe where I washed the grime and anxiety away. Then I climbed on to one of the top bunks and slept as I had never slept before. With a patient as sick as ours, none of us expected to get much rest, night or day, but for the best part of seven hours Singh Maan slept like a child, and we all seemed to wake up together just after six o'clock.

Through the Plains

As soon as I gained my bearings I had a look at the patient. His pulse was astoundingly steady, and he smiled at me.

'Still fussing about that?' he asked in clear English.

'Got to do my job', I replied. 'I'm still on duty, and you are still a long way from home.'

'Not so far – not so far now', he murmured.

At 9 a.m. the Frontier Mail pulled into the fair-sized town of Ratlam, which appeared like an oasis in the desert. This was its first respite since Bombay, and the stop lasted well over an hour. Every part of the train was checked, and wheels were systematically tapped.

The carriages were besieged with sweetmeat-sellers, trinket-sellers and sweepers all jockeying with each other for the four annas' worth of business for cleaning us out. The native population seemed poorer and more ragged than in Bombay, and the dirt and flies were as much in evidence as ever. I got out of the train, negotiated the purchase of a new ice block, and asked the coolies to bring it to the compartment. Then came the business of tipping out the old block and installing the new one, all accompanied by much shouting and pushing. I kept well out of the way.

We now faced one of the most boring stages of the journey. The land was flat and empty, no more than scrubland. The occasional villages were pathetic in their poverty, the few cows and bullocks starved and mangy. The stark problems which had faced India through the centuries seemed to stare back at me across the pitiless plain. Depressed, I tried to find diversion in the magazines we had brought with us, but the affluent advertisements only depressed me more.

By lunchtime it was suffocating, and the fans seemed to make no impression at all. Chota Lal had returned to the servants' car at the breakfast stop, so there was a little more room to move, but Hill was in a bad mood and snarled at Morgan over the desultory game of cards they were trying to play.

At 1 p.m., exactly on schedule, the train pulled into Kotah. This was a shorter stop and I went to the dining-car for a meal, having first organized the orderlies in fetching their own food. Several English passengers were in the dining-car, but I was more interested in a Sikh major sitting at the next table. He was introduced to me as Gurum Singh, and as we sat over coffee he said to me:

'I hear you have a fellow-countryman of mine in your charge, Sister.'

I guessed that the news must have reached him through the servants' quarters. I told him the story of Singh Maan, and as the train drew into a halt he asked if he could visit him.

It was now nearly half past three, and I expressed anxiety that Gurum Singh might get stuck in our compartment for several hours, for the next official stop wasn't until six o'clock.

'No, no', he said. 'I know this line. There's a whistle stop at

Kalaghari just before five o'clock. The driver's brother lives there and he pops supplies into him.'

So, together with Gurum Singh, I returned to our compartment. Singh Maan was hot and fidgety, and Morgan was bathing his head with cold swabs of gauze. After the coolness of the air-conditioned dining-car, the air seemed to carry the heat like a living thing. I felt a pang of conscience at having left Singh Maan to sweat and suffer, but the look on his face when he saw a brother Sikh was very touching. After the traditional Sikh greetings Gurum Singh sat quietly beside the dying man for the best part of an hour. There was obviously complete understanding and sympathy between the two men. Towards the end of his visit Gurum Singh braided Singh Maan's hair with rapid, practised skill. He then flicked and twisted the straggling beard into a neat strand lying under the chinline.

'There', he said, straightening up. 'You are now once more a true Sikh.'

A little later, at 6 p.m., the Frontier Mail pulled in to Muttra, by far the largest city so far. I shrieked with fright as a hairy arm snatched at me from the top of the open door. Monkeys! There were dozens of them swarming all over the train, and they had obviously been awaiting its arrival with the same avidity as the sweepers, the water-sellers and the traders. They were small and grey, and swung on to the train from the surrounding trees, yelping and barking and adding to the usual noise and confusion. This was a lighter-hearted place, whose people were better fed and more prosperous than any we had seen since Bombay.

After a while my attention was caught by the appearance of one of the pedlars, who had pretty things on a tray slung from a ribbon round his neck. His costume was colourful, striped and gay, his turban bedecked with peacock feathers. He smiled at me gently, but did not press his wares. Without thought for selection I picked out a string of turquoise beads from the tray, but he turned away and was gone before I could pay. I was still twisting the beads in my hand when Chota Lal came elbowing his way towards me along the platform.

'Sister miss-sahib', he called. 'Here good place for tea.'

'Not bazaar tea?' I queried warily.

'No, no, no', he shook his head vigorously. 'Pukka char wallah here. Good stuff. Come from north. You give one rupee. I get tea for everybody.'

It proved to be some of the finest tea I had tasted since my arrival in India. Chota Lal sat on the steps of the compartment grinning with glee at the success of his purchases. Singh Maan, watching us, smiled wanly as the train moved off into the sunset of the second day of our adventure. . . .

We drew into Delhi, the capital of all India, at 10 p.m. It was the end of the journey for Gurum Singh, who came to say goodbye. He arrived at the same time as a remarkably handsome Sikh youth of about eighteen. Gurum Singh spoke to him, then he said, 'Sister, this is Singh Maan's nephew, Achim Singh.'

The boy gave the customary bow. 'How do you do, Sister', he said in faultless English. 'I believe you have been most kind to my uncle. May I extend the heartfelt thanks of all our family.'

I suddenly felt dirty and untidy. 'Please come in', I stammered.

Hill was outside seeing about more ice, and after a meaningful nudge which failed to register, I literally hauled an equally dirty and untidy Morgan out of the train after me. Some way along the platform we found Hill. There was no sign of any ice.

'As far as I can make out,' Hill said, 'we don't shove off from here till after midnight. The ice wallahs come on shift about half past ten, so I s'pose till then we just bloomin' melt!'

'Well, we've got plenty to do', I replied wearily. 'First of all I must try to see if there's a medical officer around.' I looked at my crumpled skirt and dusty shoes. 'And I think baths all round must be on the agenda, too.'

After about ten minutes we wandered back to the compartment. Gurum Singh was saying a final goodbye. As he came out he said, 'Do you think he will make it, Sister?'

'I honestly don't know', I replied. 'He has tremendous will-power – and morphia is not only a drug, it sometimes acts almost like a food. I think perhaps that alone will get him there.'

Gurum Singh looked at me and smiled broadly. 'How old are you, Sister?' he asked.

I felt the bristles rising. This was the second time in two days that a senior officer had asked me my age. But this time I didn't feel quite so young, and the elderly Sikh officer, whose valour had earned him the distinction of a double VC, had on his face the affectionate smile of a father for a favourite daughter. I couldn't be angry.

'Twenty-four', I answered.

He didn't laugh as the major had in Bombay. Instead he placed a hand on my shoulder and said, 'It's not the morphia that will get him there, it's you. He has been living on your strength. I have seen it more than once on a battlefield. War is like that. Life is like that. We are often called on to give our strength to others. Your strength will carry him the rest of the way. . . . And now goodbye, Sister, and good luck!'

After he had gone I suddenly felt very alone. I was so lost in thought that at first I didn't realize a young British captain was speaking to me.

'I beg your pardon?' I said.

'I'm Captain Myers, Sister', he said, smiling. 'The RTO's adjutant. We've had a signal about you and your party from Bombay, and I have been assigned to you as aide while you are in Delhi. Please tell me how I can help.'

I couldn't answer for a minute, for I was too near to tears. Then as the burden lifted I came to life again. I told him some of the things I might need, and he agreed to have them sent up to me.

About ten minutes after the rest of them had gone, Achim Singh came out of the compartment. He told me he was travelling first-class, but would sit with his uncle whenever the stops were long enough.

Some while later I had a very good chicken curry and a long-awaited bath. Rested and refreshed, I returned to the platform and came to the conclusion I had got the wrong one. The front of the Frontier Mail just wasn't there. I turned to find a way out again, then panic seized me as I remembered the words of the major back in Bombay: 'The Frontier Mail divides at Delhi.' Divides!

Frantically I ran back on to the platform and clutched the first British arm I could find, which belonged to a staff sergeant.

'Where's the rest of the train?' I gasped.

'Up the line, Sister', he replied in a Scots accent.

'*Up the line*', I shrieked. 'B-b-but I've got a party on that . . . my p-p-patient. . . .'

The sergeant began to laugh. 'Oh! It's no gone for good an' all', he said.

It appeared that the centre of the train had been shunted off to be coupled to the Calcutta Express. Then it was found that they had got the wrong bit, so back came the gangs to take the train to pieces all over again. Apparently things were now well under control – as well as they ever are in India – except for the fact that the very front of the Frontier Mail, our bit, was about two miles up the line.

'It should be back any minute now, Sister', the sergeant concluded.

In spite of this alarming hiatus 'our bit' pulled out on schedule just before midnight. We now faced our second night in the train, and I took the first watch. Morgan was to relieve me at 2 a.m., and I mused half-asleep in the chair until he nudged me gently, and I turned in.

Sut Sree Akal!*

It must have been some time after 3.30 a.m. when a violent tugging at my sleeve woke me. It was Morgan.

'He's coughing blood bad', he whispered.

I was off the bunk in a leap. Hill was cradling Singh Maan in his arms. I looked at the mound of bright red swabs which had been thrown into the kidney dish on the floor. 'When did this start?' I demanded. 'You should have called me at once.'

'Only about ten minutes ago, Sister. We didn't want to disturb you till we had to. We thought it might peter out like last time.'

Singh Maan coughed again violently, the sweat pouring down his face. He clutched my hand in fear and agony. *Hamara s asa hai*', he said. ('This is my punishment.') I tried to soothe him, and wiped his forehead. '*Hamara . . . zindagi . . . bund . . . hai!*' ('My life is finished.') He was speaking in Urdu, not Punjabi, so I knew roughly what he was saying.

'No, no! This is nothing. You are not going to die *now*', I almost shouted at him.

He relaxed his grip on my hand.

'Quick! Get the ice bag out of the hold-all', I said to Morgan. 'Take these.' I handed him my scissors. 'Chip off small pieces from the ice block and fill the bag.'

The haemorrhage lasted for the best part of an hour. But that fantastically determined heart kept going through it all, and finally, with the aid of the ice and morphia, the bleeding was controlled. The next enemy was shock. We had placed Singh

Maan in a half-recumbent position, which, though it reduced the risk of further coughing, would do nothing to minimize the effect of shock. However, his condition was so extreme that it seemed advisable to leave him as he was and hope for the best.

When we at last relaxed our efforts, the dawn mists were already drifting across the Punjab. The dawn was beautiful that day – blue and mauve and saffron. Showers of birds flew up from the lush trees as the roar of the train disturbed them. As the light grew stronger they proved to be small parakeets with brilliant red and green plumage.

Singh Maan was still in a state of shock, and his hands and feet were cold. Then I remembered we had a flask of tea untouched from the night before.

'Hill', I said. 'Empty out the ice bag and put the tea in it, please.'

We placed the warm bag under the Sikh's feet, and slowly chafed his cold limbs, but he showed no signs of recovering. He lay limp and cold, like a broken doll. There was nothing for it but to use the brandy supplied by the RTO's adjutant in Delhi. If it roused him there was the risk of further haemorrhage, but I had no choice. As the train slowed down for the breakfast stop, I trickled the first of the brandy into his slack mouth. I had some difficulty in making him swallow. Then the Frontier Mail obliged by jerking itself to a halt at Jullundur. The brandy slopped over the Sikh's face. He gulped and swallowed, and for the first time stirred. As I poured some more brandy into his mouth, he groaned and coughed. Then he opened his eyes and tried to smile. I grew alarmed, thinking he was already seeing heavenly hosts, until I saw Achim Singh who had crept into the compartment, unnoticed by us.

'We've had a terrible night. Don't touch him, please, he's very weak', I said.

The young Sikh nodded, then bent towards his uncle in the traditional salaam.

Outside, Chota Lal came up with a tray of hot food. We sat on the steps of the compartment and ate ravenously. As I munched my third wheat cake, Chota Lal said:

'Sister sahib, you give white frock. Good dhobi here. Six annas.'

Suddenly I remembered the crumpled relic of a white frock which I would have to wear when we disembarked at Amritsar.

'My goodness, yes! But hurry up, you haven't got much time.'

I wandered off along the platform. The air was refreshingly cool, and the slight breeze which blew brought with it a whisper of the great hills to the north. For a long moment I looked out across the green plains. Then I walked slowly back towards the compartment. As I drew near I heard the guard blowing his whistle. I began to hurry, then I saw that Hill was still on the platform, scanning the crowd. I ran the last few yards as the guard blew the final whistle. I now knew the cause of Hill's anxiety. Chota Lal! As the train began to move, there was still no sign of him. Then we saw him, running like a greyhound.

'He'll never make it', I gasped.

But the performance he put up would have done credit to an Olympic athlete. The two orderlies heaved him in and he lay sprawled on the floor, speechless and panting, but still clutching the precious white frock, duly dhobied. I am sorry to say that our reaction was not one of gratitude, for he had given us all such a fright. Still, it was to prove the last crisis of the journey.

It was nearly noon as we steamed slowly into Amritsar. Though weary almost to the point of weeping, I arrayed myself in the 'good white frock' and a fresh cap. For the first time since leaving Poona I felt like a nurse again. The train drew to a halt, and I was the first to jump down from the compartment. A small group of Sikhs, members of Singh Maan's family, stood waiting. They were extravagantly grateful to us. With them were two white-coated figures, one of whom came forward.

'Good morning, Sister', he said. 'I am from the civil hospital. I can take charge of your patient now.'

Hill, who was standing close behind me, shifted his weight from one foot to the other. 'Just a minute', he said. 'Not so fast. We've brought him a long way, you know. I think me and me mate can just about manage to carry 'im out now we're 'ere!'

I left him to deal with the transport arrangements and went back to Singh Maan. I felt for the pulse at his wrist. The great, sunken eyes opened slowly, and fixed their gaze on my face. He knew me. I smiled at him.

'You are home, my friend', I whispered. 'Home!'

*The traditional Sikh greeting and farewell, meaning 'God is Truth'

WEAR AND CARE - METALS

Muriel Clark on choosing and caring for saucepans and cutlery

In spite of its name, I have discovered that stainless steel can be marked if you put foods like tomatoes or baked beans or anything containing tomato acid into pans and dishes made from it. Special stainless steel cleaner or soap-filled pads are the best thing to clean it with, and they usually take the marks off quite easily.

There are two stainless steel finishes available. If you're buying stainless steel vegetable dishes or tableware, for example, you can have a very shiny mirror finish; I find it difficult to keep shiny, however, and it tends to get a little scratched on the surface. Or you can get a matt finish, which I think is better. I've seen stainless steel sinks with a textured finish, which looks most attractive and prevents the drainer showing all those nasty little water marks.

Stainless steel for saucepans is usually mirror-finish, and of course they have to be mirror-finished inside. If you're buying a stainless steel saucepan, remember that it's better to have a different metal on the base because stainless steel is not a very good conductor of heat, so a heavy aluminium or copper base makes it a more efficient pan.

Personally I am very fond of the good old aluminium pans, particularly if they've got a really heavy machined bottom, because their heat conductivity is very good indeed. They don't look as nice on your kitchen shelf as a gleaming row of copper or stainless steel ones, but for cooking they're very good. A word of warning: a lot of people tend to think that the best cure for burnt food in a pan is to throw in a handful of washing soda and some water and let it soak. While this is fine for an enamel pan, you must never do it to an aluminium one because it will dissolve the metal. So first identify your saucepan, then let it soak, but not with washing soda nor with a biological detergent, either, because most of these detergents contain soda. If aluminium pans do get stained because you've boiled eggs in them or steamed a pudding, rhubarb or apple peelings boiled in them will take away that black discoloration. In soft water areas, such as where I live in Scotland, the acidity of the water tends to cause very severe pitting in aluminium – another point to consider when buying pans.

Brass and copper pans are now mostly used only for ornamental purposes in the home, and the ones in the shops have a lacquered finish. They're usually labelled accordingly, so don't clean them with commercial brass or copper polish, because you'll clean off the lacquer. All you need to do is wash them and polish them up gently. If you've got the antique variety, however, you'll have to use a commercial polish for them. Actually lemon juice and salt are considered quite good, but with the price of lemons I'd go for the polish. And, if you get tired of polishing antique pans, you can lacquer them too. You can try using a long-term polish, but if you live in an industrial area you may find that it doesn't last very much longer than the ordinary kind. If you have antique copper pans, do make sure that they are properly tinned inside, since some foods fieact with copper and may cause poisoning.

I think a table set with silver really does look most attractive; most people who have silver cutlery, as opposed to any other metal, in fact have silver plate, although they talk about it being silver. The best way to look after your table silver is to use it fairly often. Don't pack it away in its canteen and take it out only on Christmas Day; use it fairly regularly, for dinner parties, and occasionally for the family. Regular washing does cut down the amount of time you need to spend on more complicated cleaning because it stops tarnish building up. The silver plating is bound to wear off after a number of years, of course, but good-quality plate is guaranteed for something like twenty-five years' regular use.

One thing to be careful about is using a dip-type cleaner, which can affect knife handles, for example, if you let it get on to them. It's not terribly good for table silver, except to remove tarnish; I sometimes dip forks in quickly if they've got a bit of yellow from some kind of sauce or from egg. It doesn't, however, give you the same lustrous quality that polishing silver with a paste or liquid cleaner does.

ICE CREAM

Mary Berry finds this the perfect ice cream to make at home. It is rich and creamy, and many different ingredients can be used to vary the basic recipe. It needs no whisking during freezing, goes into the freezer thick and creamy, and just needs to be frozen and solidified. The quantities here serve six to eight

BASIC RECIPE

4 eggs, separated
4 oz (125 g) caster sugar
½ pint (300 ml) whipping cream
vanilla essence (optional)

Whisk the egg yolks in a small bowl until well blended. In a larger bowl whisk the egg whites with a hand rotary or electric whisk on high speed until they are stiff, then whisk in the sugar a teaspoonful at a time; the whites will get stiffer and stiffer as the sugar is added. Whisk the cream until it forms soft peaks and then fold it

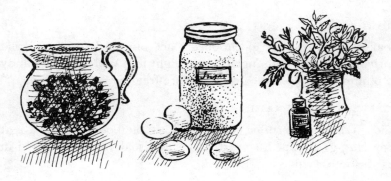

into the meringue mixture with the egg yolks. Add a little vanilla essence if liked. Turn the mixture into a 2½ pint (1.5 l) container, cover, label and freeze. Before eating, leave to thaw at room temperature for 5 minutes, then serve in scoops in small glasses or dishes.

AMERICAN MINT

Add half a bar of crushed seaside rock to the ice cream before freezing. It gives a lovely crunchy texture with pink specks.

FRESH MINT

Add a handful of finely chopped mint (chopped with a little caster sugar) before freezing.

ORANGE CHOCOLATE CHIP

Add about 2 oz (60 g) broken chocolate orange sticks before freezing.

TOFFEE BUTTERSCOTCH

Add about 4 oz (125 g) crushed butterscotch before freezing.

RASPBERRY, STRAWBERRY OR GOOSEBERRY

Use double cream and stir in ¼ pint (150 ml) fruit purée to the ice cream just before freezing. Add a little colouring if necessary.

PINEAPPLE

Use double cream. Cut the flesh from a small pineapple, add the juice of a small lemon and 2 oz (30 g) icing sugar, and purée in a blender. Then freeze until just set and fold into the ice cream just before freezing.

TUTTI FRUTTI

Soak about 4 oz (125 g) chopped glacé pineapple, raisins, dried apricots, cherries and angelica overnight in 4 tablespoons brandy to plump them up. Fold in just before freezing.

COFFEE, RUM AND RAISIN

Add 2 tablespoons coffee essence and 3 tablespoons rum to about 4 oz (125 g) chopped, stoned raisins and soak overnight. Fold in just before serving.

LIFE WITH SEVERELY HANDICAPPED CHILDREN

Dafydd and Elinor Wigley talk about the physical and emotional aspects, the difficulties and compensations

For the last six years Dafydd Wigley, MP for Caernarfon, and his wife Elinor, a professional harpist, have known that two of their four children are dying from a rare genetic disease. Both parents are carriers, although neither of them knew this until the children's disease was diagnosed when the eldest was three. There is no cure. From the age of six Alun and Geraint have progressively deteriorated, both physically and mentally. They can no longer speak, and even the simple act of moving their limbs is becoming more difficult. They are the innocent victims of an illness that affects fewer than fifty children in Britain. The reality of the children's worsening condition forces painful decisions. Dafydd and Elinor have now placed Alun and Geraint in a special hostel for five days a week. Soon the children will have to be hospitalized. The decision to lengthen the periods when they are away from home is a deliberate one intended to cushion the parents, and particularly the two younger children, from the hurt of a sudden break-up of the family. The family comes together again at the weekend.

When the Wigleys talked to *Woman's Hour* one Sunday, the two younger children were outside playing. Inside Elinor introduced Alun and Geraint, aged nine and eight. They were very aware that there was a stranger in the house, but the response was a silent one. Their father was back from Westminster, where he had been devoting much time to his Private Member's Bill to help the disabled. However, his public involvement with the disabled does not make his family's problems any easier to come to terms with, as he explained.

'I think the greatest trauma obviously comes at the very start. In our case I learned of the handicap that our two elder boys have about a week before the 1974 General Election was called, and that was when I was first elected. It was therefore a particularly difficult time, adjusting not only to the condition of the two boys, but also to a new life and new family responsibilities. It's something that weighs on my mind, but it lands even more on my wife, in that she's at home most of the time and I'm backwards and forwards between London and my constituency. When I'm at home, at the weekends, I still don't have all my time to myself. There are constituency surgeries, meetings and so on. I try to keep Sundays as free as I can for the family. Alun and Geraint are at home with us at weekends, so that they will be pottering around. They have very little or no vocabulary now – they did have up to a hundred or a hundred and fifty words at one stage, but deterioration has set in, so communication is more difficult. But one tries to spend time with them, and also with the other two of course, kicking a ball round or whatever'.

Elinor said: 'It's lovely having a reunion every week – if not every other weekend. We have a very good girl who used to live here with us. She comes back to help us every other weekend when the boys are home, because the amount of work involved is rather too much for one person, to be honest – to run a home and the four children, and cater for the special needs of the two handicapped ones. It is a particularly happy time having everybody here. As Dafydd was saying, communication is nil. They can't understand anything – no verbal direction at all, so they have to be taken physically wherever needs be. They're both doubly incontinent, and they can be a danger to themselves in many ways since they have no idea what is physically dangerous. They can't really walk very well now. So there's an awful lot of washing and looking after and caring, and also a lot of love because they are very affectionate children. They bring out a lot of love, and you feel that you want to give them a lot of love and attention. There's no aggression, nothing of the nastiness of normal children or normal people. They have just the very good qualities, without the others.'

Had they been told how long the children might live?

'No,' said Elinor, 'only in very general terms, but that is something that I'd rather not think too much about. We just enjoy them all and take it as it comes.'

When they married, did they have any idea at all that they were carriers of this disease?

'No, not at all, neither of us', said Elinor. 'It was something that we didn't know until Alun was almost three, and it came as a complete and utter shock. The doctors said the children's prognosis was rather bleak, that the length of time that they would be alive would be very short, and that there would probably be a lot of work for us. At the time it just felt that life was coming to an end. When Alun and Geraint were being diagnosed in the University Hospital in Cardiff I was already pregnant with our third child, and we were very afraid that the baby I was carrying would be affected with the same condition. I had to go through all the tests, and at the same time the doctors said if it's a little girl you'll be all right, because they thought then that Alun and Geraint had

Hunter's syndrome, which affects only boys. A year later we had another diagnosis which confirmed that they had mucopoly-sacceroidosis, but in fact a different strain of that which is called San Filippo syndrome. That can also affect girls, so the fact that she was a girl didn't automatically render her unaffected. We were very, very relieved that it was a girl – we still thought it was Hunter's syndrome then – and that when she was born she was perfectly normal. This really gave us hope and faith to look forward to the future.

'Eluned is now almost seven, absolutely full of life and enthusiasm for living. She's meant a great deal to both Dafydd and myself and her attitude is becoming very caring, I think. When she was not quite five one little incident occurred which I'll never forget. Geraint was then much more able than he is now. He was quite a naughty, mischievous little boy and he used to speak quite a bit. He did something that was probably naughty, and I thought I ought not to differentiate too much between the children, so I gave him a little row – not much, but something which I think I should have done under the circumstances. Eluned turned on me and said: 'No, no, no, no, you mustn't give Ger a row. Really, you can't. It's all right – I don't mind, you know.'

Why had they decided to have a fourth child?

'Eluned was one and quarter or so,' said Elinor, 'and she really was too important to us. We were so afraid, really, if anything should happen to her. I feel now and I felt then that she needed company. Now of course we know the decision was absolutely right, because the little boy, Hywel, is quite a character and he helps her. They're company for each other; otherwise I think she'd have been too precious.'

By the time that Elinor was having the third child doctors were able to carry out tests, and presumably those same tests would have been available when she was expecting Hywel. If it had been proven that Hywel, too, could have been a sufferer from this disease, what would she have done?

'I don't think any woman would face a termination with happiness, but to me personally, and also to Dafydd, I think, there would have been no choice but to have one.'

A great many women, faced with Elinor's situation, would probably not have been able to come to terms with it. How did she manage?

'I don't know whether I came to terms with it – I don't think one can really do that. One can, I suppose, find other things to help one along, like having the other children, and having other interests. I think basically, deep down, one never really can in any way accept it. One can try and get along, as it were, and I think we have done that so far anyway. I don't know what will happen in the future.'

'One has to live from day to day and from week to week', Dafydd said. 'I have often hankered for a visit to the United States, and I know my wife would like to go and play the harp over there, and perhaps do a tour, but these things are virtually impossible because one doesn't know what the boys' condition is going to be like.'

How important was the harp to Elinor?

'Oh, vital. If there wasn't any music, I can't think there would be an awful lot left. It's so much a part of myself, and I often feel that my heart is an extension of my hands in a way. Without it you might as well chop off my hands. I think my teaching especially has been a great help, although I would never have thought so. I'm still rather loath to admit it sometimes, because I'm not really a teacher, but it has taken me out of the house during the last seven years for about a day every week to the University in Bangor. It has been a great blessing just to be able to go out and think that for this period I'm not mother or wife or whatever, just me, and that I'm teaching these people. It has steadily increased from about two hours a week at the beginning until now I have about two days' teaching, which is as much as I want.

'I like singing, too, because I feel it is the most natural way of expressing one's feelings. I wish I could create on the harp a long vibrato sound to express what I feel – like you can on a cello or a violin – but you can't do that sort of thing with the harp. With singing, however, you can. It's such a personal thing. I'm not a professional singer, but I've enjoyed singing very, very much. The main thing for me is the response I've got from the children. Very often when we can't get any response at all from either Alun or Geraint with words, and can't even get them to look at our faces, I will start to sing. Immediately a little smile comes through and Alun will try to pronounce the words, though it's been well over a year since he's been able to say anything. He can still make the shapes of the words with his mouth. It's quite fascinating, I think, the way music appeals and gets through to people who are very handicapped.

'Before I had Alun and Geraint I took so many things for granted – being able to walk, being able to talk. It's something that you can do and that's it. However, being able to communicate by talking is a basic thing that *not* everybody can do. If people have to face being told that their child will be handicapped in the future, I would like to say to them that it's not the end of the world; there are joys to be had, a great deal that you can learn and a lot of love to be shared.

BRIAN RIX

Associated for thirty years with Whitehall farce, Brian Rix now plays a different role as Secretary-General of MENCAP, the National Society for Mentally Handicapped Children and Adults. He and his wife, actress Elspet Gray, have a mentally handicapped daughter

Our first child, Shelley, now in her late twenties, was born with Down's syndrome – in other words a mongol baby. I imagine it is just as dreadful whether it is your first, second or tenth child, because, as every parent of a mentally handicapped child will tell you, the shock is so intense. The thoughts that crowd in on you are so varied and so unfortunate and so unhappy – you're angry, you're despairing, you're worried, you have no feeling of solidarity any more. Your legs have been taken away from underneath you. As a father, I wondered what I would be able to do for my child. As a husband I was angry for my wife, because I thought it was wrong – why should it happen to her?

I was sent for by the gynaecologist to his rooms in Harley Street, because he daren't tell me in the hospital. He just said, 'Have you heard of mongolism?' and that was in a sense the end of the conversation; from then on, of course, I knew exactly what he was saying. He then asked if I would tell Elspet. When I walked into her room next day, however, Elspet had already got a pretty good idea of what was going on. I didn't have to say anything; she just took one look at me. Then a paediatrician visited Elspet and used the most appallingly inappropriate expression. Having examined

Shelley, he said, 'I'm happy to tell you your daughter is a mongol.' What he meant was, 'I'm satisfied your daughter is a mongol', but he didn't actually use those words.

Unfortunately, even a generation later, many parents still have the wrong people telling them in the wrong way. It is so prevalent even now that I am thinking of trying to organize a conference with senior members of the medical and nursing professions to see if we can't sort out how the news should eventually be broken to a mother and father. I don't think that doctors and nurses really have enough specific training in dealing with mental handicap. I'm not talking about the people who train for a career in mental health care; but I believe that during standard training doctors and nurses have something like three lectures on the cause and effect of mental handicap. This, in my view, is not enough.

Shelley lives at a special hospital – a term which, I'm glad to say, is now being dropped – called Normansfield, and comes home most weekends when we're at home. She sometimes watches me on *Let's Go*, a television programme for the mentally handicapped which I have presented from time to time. When I'm sitting beside her she will point at me on the programme and say, 'That's my Dad.' Then I say, 'Yes, but *I'm* your Dad', and she gets slightly confused. But she's sweet about it. I think the BBC are marvellous for showing these programmes round the regions, as they have.

Although I'm now working for the mentally handicapped in an official capacity, ever since Shelley was born I've been heavily involved in the fund-raising side. Now I've had to learn a great deal about the other aspects, such as welfare, politics, education, rights, social services and local authorities' responsibilities. My experience in theatre administration was to some extent helpful, I found, because administration is basically the same whether it's in the theatre or connected with work for the mentally handicapped. Fund-raising is very important because – let's face it – without money we can't finance research, in fact we can't do anything. The greatest thing we could achieve in MENCAP would be to render ourselves unemployed, because that would mean there would be no more mentally handicapped children being born. Unfortunately this is pie in the sky at the moment, but there is definitely no question that within, say, thirty years, if we were given the right financial backing and the right resources, the instance of mental handicap could probably be halved.

EPILEPSY

Sue, a mother of two, is an epileptic. She and her young son and daughter explain how they cope

Sue has epileptic fits three or four times a month, and she rarely has more than a few seconds' warning when one is coming on. She may be out shopping, walking the children to school, by herself, or with the children at home. She has had to stop being surprised at the degree of misunderstanding with which her epileptic fits are generally greeted by strangers, though there have been times when even Sue has been shocked and distressed at the treatment that she has received. 'I remember one particularly nasty incident', she said, 'when I was with Oliver in a taxi in the pouring rain. The taxi driver turned round – he heard "goings on", as he put it. Oliver was very little at the time, and he just kept saying, "Mummy, Mummy." The driver immediately assumed that I was drunk and disorderly, and said, "I'm not having drunks in my cab." With that he opened the door and put both Oliver and myself, still in the fit, out in the middle of the road in the pouring rain. The thing that occurred to me afterwards was this: supposing I had been drunk, what a place to leave a drunken woman and a toddler – in the pouring rain, in the middle of nowhere, in the street, completely unattended. What sort of man was that?'

Sue's small children, on the other hand, can certainly be counted on to be helpful – in particular the elder one, Oliver, now nine. He described what he would do when his mother was having a fit. 'I run and get a towel, and I put it not *in* her mouth, because she can't breathe then, but just at the corner. When she has little fits I'm not frightened, but occasionally I am a bit frightened.' And since Sue takes long walks to and from her children's school each day, they have often been with her in the street when she's had a fit.

'Yesterday when my Mum had a fit,' said Oliver, 'she had one of her worst ones. Strangers were coming along, and there were cars, and every car stopped to see what had happened, and I said, "Look, no need for you to start fussing. My Mum's having epilepsy." ' This is one of Oliver's most pressing tasks, to get across to people what's going on, and how, if at all, they can help. 'I tell them that my Mum has epilepsy,' he explained, 'and that they don't have to call an ambulance, and that it's nothing to fuss about and they can just help me. Sometimes they do help, but sometimes they're busy fussing a lot. It's very, very hard to stop them fussing.' Did people actually listen to him, since he's only a nine-year-old? 'No, they don't', Oliver said. 'And they ask me questions, and some questions I can't answer because I'm busy dealing with Mum. Once I didn't have anything to put in her mouth, and she cut her lip, and she started bleeding, and that was the worst one. And there was another one when my mother had a fit in a shoe shop and they called the ambulance and everything happened. I mean, she had the fit at the right time, I must say! And those were the fussiest people I've ever met in my whole life.'

Did Oliver feel it was a big responsibility? 'Yes,' he replied, 'because at the same time as looking after my Mum I have to look after my sister. My sister cries and cries, and I don't know what to do. I try to calm her down, but she still cries and cries.' In fact, although Oliver's sister Anna, who is five, isn't quite so used to the rather unusual task of looking after her mother, even she has on occasion been known to cope extremely well.

'When Oliver and Daddy were out,' Anna explained, 'Mummy had a fit on the sofa, so I got a towel quickly and put it in her mouth.' Then she just waited.

'When I came round,' Sue said, 'I realized what had happened. Anna was sitting by my side, having coped beautifully but weeping quietly because her Mummy wasn't well. I was very reassured that she could actually do the right thing on her own.'

For the brief duration of her epileptic fit Sue is totally helpless, and in a sense totally dependent on her children, although she rarely becomes unconscious. 'The general public,' said Sue, 'when they see me in the throes of a fit, aren't aware that I can hear what they're saying. This is something that's amusing to me as I'm lying there thrashing round, and quite revealing. The sort of things that emerge are the idea that, in a way, it's my fault. The most common thing I hear is, "Oh well, she's obviously forgotten her pills", as if it's my fault that I'm having this fit and it was all quite avoidable. This is nonsense, because my type of epilepsy is not and never has been adequately controlled by medication – only helped.'

Knowing exactly what the children are having to put up with, didn't Sue feel that it was all a bit much to put upon their very young shoulders? 'I feel at times that it's quite a burden for them,' she said, 'but – and I know this will be very hard for anyone to believe – I also feel in a way that it will be a strengthening process in the end. I think they are learning a lot about human nature, and about how to deal with situations on the spur of the moment.'

It is, of course, almost impossible to assess how much, if at all, the children have been affected by having a mother who suffers from epilepsy. But apart from obvious things like not carrying them around in her arms when they were babies, and of course not going swimming with them, Sue feels that she behaves very much like any other mother. 'I think the only difference, if you like, is that they tend to worry more if I don't appear, by which I mean that, if I am five minutes fetching them from school, they immediately assume that something has happened to me – and why shouldn't they assume this, since the chances are that it has? I always make sure that I'm early, if anything, to avoid putting them through that sort of agony.' In a sense, worrying about what may or may not have happened to their mother in her absence can be more trying to Oliver and Anna than actually dealing with the situation when it does happen.

It is hard to know quite how to react in the most helpful way, especially if you haven't had any previous contact with epilepsy. Sue would very much like to see some attempt made in schools to educate children about first aid, so that they will grow up into adults who can act calmly and efficiently when confronted with conditions like epilepsy. 'I know people are frightened by it,' said Sue, 'and it certainly is frightening. But I think for that reason particularly the general public should be given some idea about how to cope, because very often my friends and acquaintances have told me that, because I had told them what to expect and how to handle it, they weren't frightened.'

What should you do if you encounter someone having an epileptic fit? Rachel Field is Chief Nursing Officer at the Middlesex Hospital in London. An epileptic herself, she has worked closely over the years with the British Epilepsy Association, explaining to the uninitiated what to do. 'Don't panic', said Rachel. 'Keep calm, but be determined to help – don't run away. Wipe off any saliva that's dripping out of their mouth, and possibly put a handkerchief between the teeth, but don't force it in. If the mouth is open, it can be done. Try to protect the patient from hitting his or her arms on any hard objects, such as chairs or tables or the pavement; you do this simply by holding the hand and going with the arm. It's a good idea if you can get behind the patient, and put their head on your knee. Alternatively, if you've got a coat, put that under their head. If you can get the patient on to their side, that is the best position. But remember that the patient may be very large and very heavy, and convulsing quite rapidly. After the fit the patient may sleep, in which case the bystander would, I hope, stay with them. When the patient wakes up, be kind, and ask if there's anything you can do for them. They will know what needs to be done from then on.'

It is of course very natural that many people who find themselves witnessing a fit will react by calling for an ambulance straightaway. But, as Oliver pointed out earlier, that is the last thing that the patient may want. Rachel explained why. 'That's because of the fuss, you see. Once admitted as an outpatient in Casualty it's very difficult to get out quickly, so if you have business or school or a social event to go to, you often miss the boat. It's extremely frustrating. I wouldn't tell people never to call an ambulance, though – I think this is a situation in which the bystander should use his or her initiative. If things are not going well and the patient's colour is bad, or if the breathing is difficult, then call an ambulance. But very often by the time you've called the ambulance the fit will be over, so it's not necessary anyway.'

A DAY IN THE LIFE . . .

Ginny Bloom is deaf, but her disability has not prevented her from leading a normal professional and social life

Ginny admits that she's not very good at getting up in the morning, so, like most of us, she needs an alarm clock – but one with a difference. 'My alarm clock is attached to a vibrating pillow about the size of a dinner plate. I don't hear anything, but it's shaking my bed. Actually I've had it for so many years that I'm becoming quite immune to it.' She starts work at ten – her office operates on Flexitime, so, within limits, she can please herself.

She lives in the heart of London, very near Oxford Street, and she also works in the centre, as a computer programmer with the BBC. Though there are buses and the Underground close by, she prefers to get to the office under her own steam. 'I normally go to work by bicycle, which is quite easy. I don't really have any problems with the traffic, even though I can't hear horns and so on. I have two hearing aids and they help me to respond to some of the noise around me. I've been cycling since I was a very small child, so I'm used to it and I'm not nervous. It was very important for me to learn to drive a car, because it is my form of communication to make contact with my friends – I don't use a telephone. According to some sources deaf drivers are supposed to be a lot safer than hearing drivers, because they use their eyes a lot more.'

Though the hearing aids help her considerably, Ginny is too deaf to hear speech, so she lip-reads when people talk to her and she does it with great skill. You have to remember to face a lip-reading person directly, not to let your face be in shadow, and not to talk too fast because that makes lip-reading much harder. How long did it normally take Ginny to get to know and read fluently the speech of a new person? 'It varies – it depends on each individual', she said. 'Some people I'll never understand because they mumble so badly.'

Her speech is excellent and well modulated. How did she manage to avoid the flat speech that many deaf people have? 'I'm quite capable of developing a flat, monotonous voice', she replied. 'It happens if I'm without my hearing aids for several days. Because I wear them to monitor my voice as well as to listen to external sounds, I can hear myself speaking. If I don't have a hearing aid on for a few days my voice eventually becomes quite flat.'

Ginny was born deaf. When she was a small child, how did her parents help her to learn to speak so well? 'By hard work', was the answer. 'When you teach an ordinary child to speak you just say "Mummy", or "This is a car", once. With a deaf child you have to say it over and over again, like a repeating clockwork machine. So nearly all my early words were taught to me by people repeating the same words over and over again, and putting my hand to their mouth to feel the vibration as the air came out. Then my parents sent me to an ordinary school rather than a school for the deaf. As I was surrounded by chatting schoolgirls I had to learn to imitate them; so, in the course of time, I acquired language.'

Ginny works in an ordinary office, writing instructions in a special code or language which will tell the computer what to do. She explained in layman's terms what programming is all about. 'A computer can't do anything unless you tell it what to do. Now let's say we want to tell the computer to make a cup of tea. You have to write a series of instructions. First question: is the stove present – yes or no? If not, acquire stove. Go back to the beginning. Is the stove present? Yes. Next question: is the kettle present – yes or no? No. Get the kettle. Now you want to put the kettle on the stove, so you ask: is the kettle on the stove? Yes. Is it filled with water? No. You write all these instructions down until finally you've got your cup of tea.'

Having written the program, Ginny feeds it into the computer. She types her instructions on a keyboard that's linked to the machine and it answers in writing too, either in a printed form or by flashing its replies up on a kind of television screen. For Ginny it's often easier than communicating with the other people in her office, but there is no real problem there because everyone takes the situation very much in their stride, including Ginny's boss, Eric Pickering. 'Problems are there to be overcome,' said Eric, 'and we overcome them. Everyone's got used to Ginny and they regard the situation now as a perfectly normal one. She's a fairly vivacious person – not difficult to get to know, anyway. Since she's outgoing, people perhaps make a greater effort to get to know her and communicate with her.'

There's one thing Ginny can't do, and that's use the telephone, at any rate not without help. However several of her colleagues are very good at helping on the rare occasions when she has to ring someone. When *Woman's Hour* talked to Ginny, Tony was acting as interpreter while she phoned a friend. Ginny spoke for herself while Tony listened on an extension and repeated the replies from the other end, so that she could lip-read them.

'Hello, Martin. Ginny here', she began. 'Tony's on the extension, listening to what you're saying. My husband, Jim, would like to speak to you about this new computer centre, and it might be an idea if we all met one evening after work.'

There was a pause, then Tony relayed Martin's reply for Ginny to lip-read, 'Sounds like a good idea.'

'What about next week?' Ginny asked. 'Monday? Wednesday?'

Another pause. 'Whichever suits you.'

'Right. Wednesday evening, then.'

'Fine.'

'Which pub do you normally call into?'

After a moment, 'Do you know the Nightingale?'

'Yes. I'll see you there on Wednesday, eight o'clock. . . .'

Clearly this system of making a telephone call worked well, since there were hardly any hold-ups in the conversation.

At lunch-time Ginny sometimes works right through, eating a snack in the office, but she likes to get out and about when she can. She enjoys the shops and restaurants of the West End, and also, as she explained, the smaller back streets behind the tourist area. 'I try, if I'm not too lazy, to get down to Berwick Street Market, which I love because there's so much action, so much to see. I just shop and watch people arguing and laughing. It's a completely different world from walking along Oxford Street, which is full of tourists – they're a boring bunch.'

Back in the office once more, Ginny works until about six and then goes home to her flat to make supper for herself and her husband. She enjoys cooking and entertaining; the next day they had eight people coming to dinner, so she spent some of the evening preparing for that. Ginny met Jim, a Post Office engineer, some years ago, and he takes her deafness without fuss, as a matter of course. Ginny described their relationship. 'When I have my down days, or a frustrating day because of my deafness, he just says, "So what? It's something you have to put up with." He didn't marry me because he felt sorry for me – in fact he said he was attracted to me because of my voice. Jim and I like each other as people, rather than for what we lack.'

Ginny and Jim often go out for an evening with friends, or to a restaurant or party. Ginny likes to be around people, but if it's too large a group she does have problems, sometimes with quite comical results. 'If I try to follow a group conversation,' she said, 'sometimes I get completely the wrong idea. I was at a party once and everybody was arguing about something. I thought I understood what they were saying and jumped in and said, "No, I don't think so. I think contraceptives should be so-and-so!" Everybody stopped talking and looked at me. They weren't in fact talking about contraceptives, but about contact lenses!'

Ginny has learnt how to handle the consequences of her deafness, and even on those days when things are frustrating rather than funny her basic approach is the same – to put her handicap firmly in its place. She spelt out her philosophy. 'I was brought up on the theory that everybody has something wrong. I used to come home from school crying and saying, "I'm deaf. Why aren't I like other girls?" My mother used to answer, "Look at Mary, she's got bad eyes. Look at Diana, she's got bad kneecaps. Look at Clare, her father's dead. Everyone's got something wrong, and no one is perfect. They've all got a worry of some kind." When I was younger I blamed my ears for everything – if I fell over and hurt my ankle, say, or if I didn't seem to have any friends. But later I realized it had nothing to do with my ears – it was my personality.'

PATRICK NUTTGENS

Dr Patrick Nuttgens, Director of Leeds Polytechnic, trained as an architect. He has appeared in a number of television programmes on buildings and the environment

When I was leaving school and thinking about where I might go to study I actually turned down the possibility of a place at Cambridge – that is almost unique, by the way, as a sign of incipient lunacy. Eventually I went to Edinburgh, which I found exciting and dramatic, but it never crossed my mind that I would ever go to a city or town that wasn't beautiful to look at, because that's part of my background. So to go to Leeds was indeed a shock. However after ten years there, at first working there and living outside, and now also living inside Leeds, I find it more and more exciting and rewarding as a place to examine. It is *the* great paradigm of an industrial city. It also has that fantastic town hall which is the very symbol of the grandeur, arrogance and sheer bloody-mindedness of local government in the mid-nineteenth century. I love Leeds now, and I really enjoy working there because they're very nice people. To express it another way, when I left the university world in York and went to the polytechnic world in Leeds I remember saying to somebody, adapting a phrase which I think is BBC, that whereas in the university world people occasionally stabbed you in the back, in Leeds they always stabbed you in the front. They have stabbed me several times, by the way, but I quite like it really.

It was in fact more of a shock giving up being a university professor than it was moving from York to Leeds. To give up being a professor really means writing yourself off in society. I have practised as an architect, though only in a small way. You can't teach architecture properly – nor can you teach any subject in my view – unless you are involved in the activity which you are teaching. Therefore I've always done and still do a small amount of architectural work. The first thing I ever did was a belltower for a church in Mallaig, which was extremely difficult because the old canon, who had taken thirty years to stop the roof leaking, wouldn't let me move a single slate. I had to put the belltower on top of the roof without moving the slates, and it was extremely difficult – but I love that.

My father, now eighty-eight, has worked in stained glass all his life and is still active; he's spent most of his life putting windows into very ordinary churches all over Britain. He took it up, almost accidentally, when he was a boy. He left school at the age of fourteen or so and got a job in an office addressing envelopes, then one in a factory, and so on. Then he discovered, when he was still very young, that he had not only a great ability to draw, but also a tremendous love of stained glass; so that since he was about twenty or so he has always worked in stained glass. He designs and makes the windows and puts them in – he does the whole job. In a sense he's the oldest surviving follower of William Morris, since he covers all the various activities and works in a very traditional way. Anybody in the stained glass world will say that my father knows more about the craft of stained glass than anybody else alive, and I think he puts that into action. But he is a very logical, orthodox, practical chap; his windows actually fit and by and large they keep the rain out, which is really very important.

The family name is originally German, but from the very borderland, from Aachen, which used to be called Aix-la-Chapelle; Nuttgens should really have an umlaut over the 'u', and be spelt Nüttgens. The family lived and still live in this border country of Germany, Holland and Belgium. Shortly after we were married my wife and I were in the south of Holland, and we crossed to Aachen and rang up everybody in the telephone directory with my name. Eventually we found somebody who spoke German sufficiently slowly for me to understand, and we discovered that we represented English, German, Belgian, Dutch, American and various other nationalities. We gathered everybody together and had a tremendous party. We crossed the border late at night trying to get back, and I think the border guards were not terribly amused. But the point is that the Nuttgenses are borderland people, of whom it is always said that whoever wins, they lose. Funnily enough, one of the things that you do if you're that sort of person is become some kind of craftsman. My father learned to be a craftsman, though he's actually an extremely good painter, and could have been a very fine portrait painter. But when I got to know all these Nüttgenses and Nootghenses I discovered that, although my father had not known it when he originally took up stained glass, in the past nearly all of them had been artists or craftsmen, beating copper and so on, but they had also been stained glass artists. That is very odd, and one wonders whether it is in the genes. The one thing that still gets me really worked up is stained glass.

I'm used to large families because I'm one of twelve sons and I have eight children of my own plus a foster-son. When I was a lad myself I contracted polio, which certainly affected what I did with my life. I was twelve and at boarding school, and I shall never forget it. I walked off a rugby pitch – I was captain of the junior fifteen – and that was the last time I ever ran in my life. I've never been able to run since then, and I've always had some kind of splint, but until the last five years nobody would really have known because I taught myself to walk sufficiently straight and to pretend to be perfectly all right, so that nobody would notice. It rules out a whole area of activity – obviously all sports as a normally active participant, though not, if I went into an orthopaedic hospital, something like polio cricket, which is an amazing game. It takes about an hour to run up to the wicket and bowl – it's tremendous fun. The effect really is more a psychological one, and I think it made me turn to academic life more quickly than someone who was physically active might have done. I remember at school somebody suggested I might be a politician, and I decided that that was really not my world – not because I wanted to be academic in the sense of not being part of things, but because I just didn't feel at home in that part of the world. I wanted to reflect about things.

Since I was fourteen I've never spent a single day without pain, and that's part of my life. I don't mind it, because I'm used to it and it's part of me. But it does give one a different view of other people. I think it makes one rather intolerant in some ways – not about oneself, but about pretentious people.

It may also influence some of my feelings about architecture. The reason for choosing architecture as my field, however, was not just the polio. I had always been fascinated by architecture, partly because my father used to take us to look at old churches at weekends. I am very intolerant about some modern architecture and I get deeply involved in it. I went off to be a student in order to become a great architect; it took me about five years to realize that, though I was competent, I wasn't all that good. But I do think we have got a lot of rethinking to do about the humanity which we ought to be injecting into it.

ART FOR THE PEOPLE

Sir Hugh Casson, an architect by training, is President of the Royal Academy of Arts. Here he puts his case for the de-intellectualization of the visual arts

I have been heard to say that the two biggest industries in Britain today are the commercialization of anxiety and the manufacture of distrust. They are not only very big, but also very successful, and that's not surprising considering how hard we all work at it. All day and every day we're told or we busy ourselves telling other people how terrible everything is and most people are. Politicians are mountebanks, we declare, industry is a conspiracy of crooks and layabouts, the police are brutal, the law corrupt, the arts a con. It's a sort of steady drip-feed of self-indulgent discontent, made even more pernicious in my view by a cult of self-absorption as tedious to others as it is unhelpful to ourselves. There's a good side to it all, of course – scepticism and self-questioning needn't do any harm. Experts become perhaps a little more humble, and non-experts get more of a say in trying to put things right. But the general effect is debilitating, and it leaves us groping around in a fog of irritable apathy in which all the old signposts seem either to have disappeared or to point in very unhelpful directions.

Among the familiar signposts, such as religion and scholarship and nature, are of course the visual arts. Once they seemed there to inspire us, to enrich and delight our lives, but for the last fifty years or so they seem to have vanished into carefully guarded museums or private studios. And when we do meet them, to be frank they're not always very easy to love. Indeed, despite the fantastic growth in technical art media, prints and lithographs, postcards and television and video, the gap between the living fine arts and the public does at times seem wider than ever. Most modern painting and sculpture to most people seems austere and solemn, perverse and aggressive and ugly, and nearly always inexplicable. Indeed you could say that most people avoid most art because most art avoids most people.

Now it's much easier to bewail this or to be irritated by it than it is to explain how and why it has happened. Obviously there are many reasons, some basic, some trivial. There's the artist's reaction from the moth-eaten sentimentality of much nineteenth-century painting, and his distaste for what seems to be the repellent commercialism and king-making of the art-dealing world; his wish to clear a clean, small space, so to speak, in a world that's absolutely swamped with images; his enthusiastic exploration of new techniques, his developing interest in the process rather than in the product. But there are other less noble influences affecting all of us, not just artists: the cult of self-expression at the expense of everything else, for instance; the dismissal of all standards as authoritarian, and all skills and disciplines as restraints upon one's spontaneity. There's the rise to power of the written word and that academic attitude which overvalues those who write and talk in relation to those who make and do. The result is that art becomes over-intellectualized and often quite unintelligible without the help of interpreters, and goodness knows they're pretty difficult to understand too. Then there's the cult of the artist as a philosopher-priest figure, a role which he doesn't mind accepting, however intellectually unable to sustain; and finally the virtual disappearance of the private patron – quirky and unpredictable, always backing his fancy with his own money – and the appearance on the scene of state patronage and all the risks of official taste.

When you empty all these disturbing and uncomfortable ingredients into that familiar old mixing bowl called British artistic taste, which – put very brutally – assumes that the arts are nothing at all to do with daily life but can safely be left to the weekend and to the wife, not surprisingly the results are often distasteful, or fail to nourish. Well, you may say, why worry? Art's old enough and powerful enough to go underground for a while, to look after itself without our support. It will survive since it is invincible. True enough. And it's certainly no good cursing the artist. He does what he must and not what he's told – hence his vulnerability to persecution in the totalitarian world, of course. His strength lies in his total single-mindedness and in the careful and often agonizing solution to his own problems and not to ours.

Nevertheless, perhaps because I've worked all my life in the world of the visual arts, though as an architect not always at the centre, I am an optimist. Of course I too get cross from time to time. I find it particularly irritating, for instance, that the qualities of imagination, creativity and skill required to design, say, a type-writer or a washing machine are not regarded by the academics as worthy of any serious study or critical assessment. But I am encouraged by the way the arts, for all their occasional silliness and pretentious self-protectionism, are continuing to thrive. And would I be over-optimistic, I wonder, to suppose that at last our over-literary educationalists are beginning to recognize that art is or can be a serious and vigorous discipline? It's not just a part-time hobby, or, to quote Sir Thomas Beecham, 'a racket run by un-scrupulous men for unhealthy women'. At last, I think, non-artists are beginning to be more visually sophisticated about what they look at and to recognize more easily the charlatan or the peacock. At last the official guardians of art, the critics, pundits, historians and museum curators, are beginning to recognize that the public would like an occasional look in as well. And at last we're recognizing that creativity is not limited to a chosen few but is available to be discovered and nourished at many levels.

THE AUSTRALIAN LIFESTYLE

People in Australia tend to live very differently from the British, as a Sydney family demonstrates, and an initiate explains how a simple, unsophisticated invention called the eskie has changed the whole face of Australian social life

'We have a lot of swimming parties in the summer,' said Bill Hayes, 'because at this time of the year the weather is great and we can enjoy the pool. It's easy to entertain people because we come outside and sit by the pool. We don't have to take people into the house, so we don't have to be conscious of worrying about the house getting mucked up and so on.' Someone mentioned something about a 'skinny dipping party'. What did that mean? 'Well,' he continued, 'later on maybe the cozzies will come off and there might be a bit of nudity – topless swimming among the girls. Depends on how much we've had to drink and how the night progresses.'

Barbara, Bill's wife, said that they entertained quite a lot, and in good weather outside, as Bill had said. 'Definitely in the back yard by the pool and with a barbecue. But if it's not nice weather we normally have it inside and have a buffet with different hot dishes.'

Australians are sociable and hospitable but they are also very private, and back yards have high brick walls separating them from the neighbours. 'We like to be able to invite our friends in and do our own thing', said Bill. 'If we want to swim and sunbathe we can do it. We also like to be private from our neighbours who we're not so friendly with.'

Barbara loved her home, she said, and it was very important to her. 'Around the house I do the cooking, shopping, washing and ironing, and because I go to work I concentrate, towards the end of the week – Friday afternoon, Saturday morning – on a good clean right through, and just do little bits during the week.' It is still the woman's role in Australian society to be the housewife, but Barbara said that Bill and their two children were a great help.

Saturday is Bill's day for doing things around the house and garden. 'I generally cut the grass, trim the hedges, hose the place down. I might paint, or I might be renovating, or I might be gardening, but I always spend all day Saturday working around the house. About four o'clock I knock off and have a couple of beers and sit with the family and we chat. Then we have a meal and perhaps watch a bit of telly. It's early to bed because we tend not to do anything on Sunday – we just relax. I might go fishing early in the morning, then come home and sit by the pool and entertain our friends or just ourselves.'

Sunday lunchtime usually means a barbecue, and that day it was the job of Murray, Bill and Barbara's son, to light it. 'I've got to lay it first,' he said, 'and stack all the wood up so it burns properly. If you just clump it in a pile air doesn't get through and it doesn't burn. Then I've got to light it.'

Bill described the kind of food they had at a typical barbecue. 'We have chops and sausages and rump steak, or a bit of topside or sirloin. What we normally do is buy a whole rump, slice it up into thick pieces, and marinade it in a Chinese barbecue sauce. We leave it overnight and it's fantastic the next day. It gets a flavour all of its own – the smoky flavour of the wood plus the barbecue sauce really turns you on.'

The beach is an important element in the life of many Australians. 'We live about three minutes' easy walk from it', said Bill. 'Just up over the hill and down to the beach. There you go!' We moved our home about fourteen, fifteen months ago to be here by the ocean. I like to get down here every afternoon after work. I work Flexitime, so I start at 7.30 and finish at 3.30. I'll be down here at 4.30 so I can spend an hour or two swimming and perhaps go out fishing or take the kids on the boat for a ride. We surf, swim, even put a face mask and snorkel on and do a bit of scuba diving just to watch the aquatic life. It's beautiful.'

The standard of living in Australia is generally higher than in Britain, but the cost of living isn't. Australia has the highest home ownership per head of population in the world. 'We had our first home when we'd been married three or four months', said Bill. 'We bought a little semi-detached cottage and sold that after eight years. Then we bought a block of land, built a home and lived in that for another seven or eight years. After that we bought this home, moving up every time. It's simple to do – you can re-finance, taking out a fresh mortgage of course, and gradually increase your lifestyle.' Lifestyle seems to be a matter of prestige and one-upmanship to Australians, which Bill confirmed. 'It's a bit of a competition between people you work with, you know –

where you live and how you live.'

The house the Hayes live in had cost them 85,000 dollars fourteen months previously. 'I think in the six months after we bought it', said Bill, 'there was a 17 per cent overall increase in values in the eastern suburbs of Sydney, and now I should say the house was worth about 115,000, maybe 120,000 dollars.' Their house would fetch, therefore, about £60,000 sterling. But this was in Coogee, one of the eastern suburbs, a fairly sought-after area, and Sydney anyway is the most expensive city in Australia. In Melbourne or the other state capitals it would be possible to buy a nice three-bedroomed house with a pool for between, say, £40,000 and £50,000. And of course salaries are higher in Australia: Bill earns 20,000 dollars a year – about £10,000 – and Barbara about 7,500 dollars. Cars are more expensive than in Britain, but all the other consumer goods are cheap enough to be considered necessities rather than luxuries. Barbara described what they had in the house.

'In the utility room we have a big, fully automatic washing machine and a dryer to go with it. There's a second fridge and a second freezer over on the other side, and a big water heater. In the kitchen there's a double wall oven and a hob, plus a big fridge, a freezer and a dish-washer. We have three televisions in the house – there's a big colour one in the lounge room, and then our daughter, Helen, has a coloured one in her bedroom and Murray has a black-and-white in his.'

'We watch a lot of television', said Bill. 'I would say at least four hours a night. I like the ABC shows, the documentaries, the imports from England and the local material, whatever it is – talk-back shows, that type of thing. I get a lot of pleasure out of it. There's never any dispute about who's going to watch what, so far as I'm concerned – the one in the lounge room's mine!'

The only night the Hayes family don't watch television is when they're having a pool party. A lot of people think that at Australian parties the women go to one end and the men to the other end. 'It does happen,' said Barbara, 'but usually we find that when they first arrive the women get together and chat about everyday things and the men talk about the races or their golf, but we all intermingle in the end.'

'I talk to everyone who is here,' said Bill, 'but we men all seem to congregate together, talking about what we've been doing that day. The talk often gravitates around whether we've had any success at the races. I have a bet every Saturday and perhaps once during the week, but there are race meetings on six days a week as well as dog meetings and trotting meetings, and people bet fairly frequently on them.'

A lot of drinking goes on at Australian parties. One of Bill and Barbara's guests said that it was the main activity, and beer was the favourite drink. How many tins did he think men consumed at a party? 'I bring about two dozen', he said. 'I usually get through them before I go home.' The beer is kept cold in a device

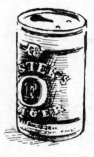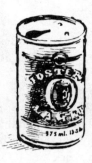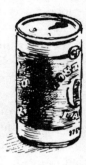

called an eskie, which is a portable ice box. It will hold four dozen cans of beer and a bag of ice, plus two things called 'chooks', a term which had to be explained by a native. 'A chook is a chicken, otherwise known as a goodchigoy, which is the staple diet of football followers and cricket fans. They'll take a couple of chooks with them if they go to the cricket ground to watch the Poms get a thrashing. The height of bad manners is to be invited to a blokes' party and not take your drink. As I drink quite a vast quantity, when I go to a party I take my eskie with me. I'll take my two dozen cans plus ice and it'll last me all night. If anything's left over I come and knock it off next morning.'

The invention of the eskie is one reason why the men and women no longer remain separate throughout parties. 'Nowadays with the use of tins and bottles, the guy is much more mobile. He whizzes up to his eskie, sticks his clammy paw into it, whips out a cold tin and he's off and racing right. Now there's no problems there. But previously the blokes would be down by the drink, and the sheilas would be down there standing around beside the flagons or sitting there having their small talk and rubbish. Nowadays the Australian male is much more mobile in his drinking because of his portable can of cold beer.'

MAYONNAISE

Mary Berry's recipe makes ½ pint (300 ml) of basic mayonnaise, and the variations can be used with lots of different dishes

BASIC RECIPE

2 egg yolks
1 level teaspoon made mustard
1 scant teaspoon salt
1 level teaspoon caster sugar
pepper to taste
1 tablespoon white wine vinegar or cider vinegar
½ pint (300 ml) oil – olive, corn or vegetable
1 tablespoon lemon juice

Cut a small wedge from an old cork, and put the cork into the neck of your oil bottle. This will enable you to add oil to the mixture a drop at a time. Stand your bowl on a damp cloth to prevent it slipping on the work surface. Put the yolks, mustard,

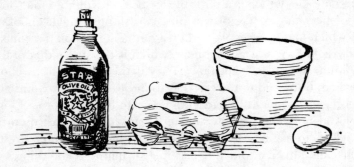

salt, sugar and pepper into a bowl with the vinegar and mix well. Add the oil drop by drop, beating well with a whisk the whole time until the mixture is smooth and thick. Lastly beat in the lemon juice.

BLENDER MAYONNAISE

Use the same basic ingredients, but add 1 large whole egg instead of the 2 egg yolks. Put the egg, seasoning and vinegar in the blender and run for 30 seconds or until blended. Remove the small cap in the lid and pour the oil into the blender in a steady stream, with the blender on a low setting. When all the oil has been added the mayonnaise will be very thick. Then add the lemon juice and blend.

VARIATIONS

Herb Mayonnaise: To the basic recipe add 1 tablespoon finely chopped parsley, 1 tablespoon finely chopped chives and a little finely chopped fresh tarragon and basil, if available. This is very good with 2 tablespoons double cream stirred in and served with fish or meat salads.

Aioli: Add 2 crushed cloves of garlic to the basic recipe.

Curry Mayonnaise: To the basic recipe add 1 level teaspoon curry powder and 2 tablespoons finely chopped mango chutney. Add the curry powder to the egg yolks.

Lemon Mayonnaise: Increase the lemon juice to 2 tablespoons or more, to taste, and omit the vinegar.

Anchovy Mayonnaise: Stir 4 tablespoons anchovy essence into the finished mayonnaise. Use in fish and vegetable salads.

Avocado Mayonnaise: Add to the basic mayonnaise 1 large avocado puréed with 2 teaspoons lemon juice, and season with lots of freshly ground black pepper.

Prawn or Shrimp Cocktail Sauce: To the basic mayonnaise add 1 level teaspoon tomato purée, a pinch of sugar, a few drops of Worcester sauce, 2 drops of tabasco and a little extra lemon juice. If you like it more piquant, add 1 tablespoon horseradish cream.

Tartare Sauce: To the basic recipe add 1 rounded dessertspoon each chopped gherkins, capers and parsley. Serve with hot fish dishes.

THOUGHTS ON NUCLEAR DISARMAMENT

Oliver Postgate is a writer and film-maker

Are you old enough to remember 1945? I remember a day in early August. . . . I was in Essex at the time. I opened the newspaper and read the headlines: ATOM BOMB DROPPED ON HIROSHIMA – MANY DEAD.

What I felt was a sort of scream inside myself, a silent scream, not easy to describe. It was pity . . . yes, pity. Pity for the many dead and for the many slowly dying. But many had died in

Stalingrad, and in the firestorm raids on cities like Dresden. At that end of the war the words 'many dead' were a familiar grief.

No, this was something else. This was a cold dread, an icy hand laid on the future, on the future of my children yet to be born, on the future of all mankind. That scream has stayed inside me ever since. I think it is somewhere inside everybody who lived through that day, and inside many who were not even born then.

The years immediately after the war passed without anybody letting any more atom bombs off. The scream grew quiet. The superpowers built up their stockpiles and stood up their rockets, but in the end they seemed to accept, almost with relief, the certainty that if either of them was to launch atom bombs against the other, they would themselves be destroyed. This was known as Mutually Assured Destruction – M.A.D. – mad!

Although it was essentially mad, that acceptance did seem to close the Pandora's Box. It was a shameful compromise which I believe has contributed and is still contributing a deep infective anxiety to the whole of society. There is a permanent question mark over all our lives . . . do we have a future? It is not easy to know exactly what effect this primal anxiety has, but I suspect it is far deeper and more serious than we realize.

However, that is how things were. It brought us the relatively quiet years of the sixties and early seventies, during which the attitudes generally held about nuclear armaments were formed. It was not essential to know the exact details of the nuclear armaments because they were, in a sense, academic – a formality – because central to the policies of all the nuclear powers was something called 'deterrence'. This was the M.A.D. acceptance – that nuclear war is essentially unthinkable. To use nuclear bombs was clearly recognized, even by politicians, as global suicide.

That is still true, but recently there have been debates, policy documents written in the elaborately coy language of nuclear carnage, demonstrations of potty air-raid precautions and discussions about life in a post-nuclear world. I have come to realize something that has brought back that scream with deafening force. Somebody, somewhere does not know that it is still true.

What has happened is that the unthinkable has officially become thinkable, and is now being presented to us in such a way as to try and persuade us that nuclear warfare is not only likely but is in some way acceptable, and that we can quietly acquiesce to it in the same way that we once acquiesced to the myth of deterrence. What has changed is that the essentially mad stalemate which used to be called deterrence was based only on the absolute assumption, shared by all, that nuclear warfare is totally unthinkable. Once it becomes thinkable, 'deterrence' simply ceases to exist. Nuclear warfare becomes, has become, what they might call a 'viable strategic option'.

Because of this, mankind now faces an unimaginably terrible danger. It is not so much the danger of the bomb itself, though that would be the instrument, but the danger of a failure of the imagination . . . the danger that we may not see the danger . . . the danger that we will share the blindness of our politicians and fail to realize fully what we are talking about.

Man has been busily inflicting inhumanity on man for thousands of years. The sum total of man's injustice, oppression, misery, pain and murder is so vast as to be uncountable. Yet one piece of arithmetic is certain – by turning two keys and pressing a button, the total of man's inhumanity to man since the beginning of time would be exceeded, probably many times over, in a few hours of what would be called 'strategic response activation' – a sort of do-it-yourself Armageddon that would burn many millions of innocent people to death in a flash, would burn many millions more to death more slowly, would condemn hundreds of millions more to a hideous lingering death, scraping for scraps in the radio-active debris of our cities, and could finally leave this planet a dead dump, a lifeless, poisoned, poisonous waste, spinning uncounted years in empty space, a place where, to all intents and purposes, the human race never happened.

To do that is now within the power of man.

To threaten to do that seems to be within the intent of man . . . indeed, it is the corner-stone of Britain's foreign policy.

About this we can ask, in fact we must ask, one simple question: 'Is there any human purpose that could be served by the extinction of the human race?' Or, come to that: 'Is there any human purpose that could be served by *threatening* the extinction of the human race?' because a threat is meaningless unless you mean to carry it out, so it comes to the same thing.

The whole human race lives every day under that threat, and under that threat our greatest peril lies in our doing nothing about it.

LONE VOYAGERS

*Margaret Hicks, a Southampton schoolteacher in her forties, became in
1980 the first woman to make a double crossing of the Atlantic single-handed
in a small boat. Geoffrey Moorhouse's travels were on land – in 1972 he
set out on a lone, 3,500-mile journey across the Sahara from west to east
with camels*

Geoffrey Moorhouse had two reasons for undertaking his spectacular journey. 'The smaller, and I suppose the less worthy of
them', he said, 'was that no one had ever before crossed the Sahara
in the old-fashioned way with camels from west to east, and I
wanted to try to do this. In other words I wanted to break a
record. I didn't succeed. The second reason, and much more
important, was that I wanted to find out what happens to a very
ordinary human being, brought up in a so-called civilized Western
society, when he's confronted with a completely alien and at times
rather hostile environment. In a way it was an attempt to debunk
the myth of the superman, because I'd read so many books about
people doing hard journeys over rough portions of the Earth and
it always seemed to me that they had left something out of their
account, or that they weren't as other men are. Most people are as
other men are – I don't believe in the superman concept and I
wanted to record accurately what it was like.'

Although, as he pointed out, Geoffrey didn't complete his crossing, he still managed to cross two thousand miles of desert, which
is very impressive. Margaret Hicks explained her reasons for setting out to cross the Atlantic twice in a small boat. 'In some ways
my reasons are very similar to Geoffrey's,' she began, 'which is
very interesting. First of all I wanted to achieve something, to do
something for my own personal satisfaction. I looked round at the
sailing records, and since no woman had made a double Atlantic
crossing in a conventional monohull, I thought I would have a
bash. And then of course it was the supreme ego-trip, if I am
going to be absolutely honest. I wanted to lift myself out of the
mass of people, to assert my individuality. I feel that today we
often get so lost in mammoth organizations such as large schools.
I've seen my pupils looking lost, as if in a crowd, and I wanted to
show that an ordinary schoolteacher could get up and do something – something that didn't cost an excessive amount of money,

but that I could achieve. And I can't tell you how pleased I am to have managed it.'

The hardest thing for Geoffrey to overcome was exhaustion. 'I became so weary, not just at the end of every day but cumulatively. The trip took about six months altogether, and after about a month it was a bit of an effort to keep going. At one point I was presented with the most frightening circumstances of all – missing a well when I'd virtually run out of water, so that it was a toss-up whether I would last another forty-eight hours. I had to do certain things if I was to survive at all, and the mere fact that I'd geared myself to this plan of action seemed to anaesthetize the fear. Being faced with the actuality of possible catastrophe wasn't nearly as bad as it was in prospect before it ever happened.'

Margaret, too, felt there were moments on these trips when she might not survive. 'In retrospect, I felt it was a very interesting experience, because I knew that the possibility of death was ever-present – but it's one thing to know it and another actually to confront it. In the initial part of the journey, crossing the Bay of Biscay, I ran into a succession of very bad gales up to Force 10; at one time I thought there was a very good chance of the boat foundering. At first I found myself almost paralyzed with fright, but I couldn't keep up this level of emotion – it was just too exhausting. Somehow the will to live, the fight to survive, took over, and I was determined that no way were the elements going to get the better of me. Therefore I embarked on Operation Survive. I said to myself that supposing the boat did founder, supposing it did sink, the end of the world wouldn't have come. I would put into operation Plan B, which meant getting into the liferaft. I then became totally preoccupied in arranging my Abandon Ship preparations, which I found, as with Geoffrey, completely anaesthetized me against fear.'

Extreme physical discomfort was obviously something that both Margaret and Geoffrey had to endure. 'It was always with me', said Geoffrey. 'I had to quit after doing a couple of thousand miles for two reasons. The first was that I got dysentery very badly and I virtually couldn't walk any further, and the second was that I'd lost so many camels. I had six altogether; I never had more than three at any one time, but I had them in relays, and of these six, three died. I had simply got to the point where I couldn't go any further. There was always physical discomfort, but after a while I became accustomed to it. In retrospect I think with amazement and revulsion about the fact that I was lice-ridden and had saddle sores for six months.'

Keeping clean was a problem for Margaret, since being on so small a boat she had to restrict her freshwater supplies exclusively to drinking and cooking. 'In fact half-way through my first transatlantic crossing', she said, 'I came to the conclusion that I had to be either stark, staring mad or a masochist to travel in such an excruciatingly uncomfortable fashion. In a small boat the motion even in slight seas is quite considerable, and one is constantly thrown all over the place. It's very difficult to do anything, and it may surprise people to know that I spent almost the entire journey across the Atlantic lying down, because there just wasn't anything else I could do. I was strapped on, because it's very easy to fall off a small boat. When I left England I put on my safety harness and I literally did not take it off, even to go to bed, until I arrived safely in Antigua.'

There must presumably have been compensations, though, such as, for Geoffrey, wonderful desert sunsets and sunrises, but he said there were fewer than perhaps he had expected because people tend to romanticize the desert. 'There were marvellous stars at night, and I could see all sorts of constellations coming up the horizon and gradually going over the sky. The trouble was that I couldn't appreciate the beauty of the desert because I was so preoccupied with the safety factor. I longed for the most trivial things – and this was one of my most astonishing discoveries, how very, very trivial one's thoughts could be. I can remember spending the best part of a day, without exaggeration, thinking how, when I got home, I would make myself cheese and onion pie. Of course, all I was eating was plained boiled rice and a bit of meat occasionally, which was damn dull. I longed for something with a bit of taste to it, as my granny would have said.'

Margaret, lying down in her small boat, had similar dreams. 'I know this sounds equally incredible, but all I could think of was a nice glass of cool, iced, fresh milk. This occupied my thoughts far more than I ever would have imagined possible, although, unlike Geoffrey, I did eat very well, because I was able to take specially prepared food packs which were very easy to prepare – I had beef stroganoff and *coq au vin* and things like that.' She found it important to give herself little treats to look forward to. 'I used to arrange special dinners – my quarter-of-the-way dinner, my half-way dinner, and my three-quarters-of-the-way dinner. Really at any excuse I could find I would have a celebration to ease up the voyage.'

On such journeys one's timescales must become quite different. 'I would have suffered far less mental anguish', said Geoffrey, 'if I had been able to adjust to the environmental timescale, which, in the case of the desert, is the day or the week or the month. But partly because I had the problem of navigation, and therefore I had a watch in my equipment, and partly because I come from a Western society in which the minute or the hour, at the very most, are the timescale, I was constantly fretting and felt a kind of friction between the actuality and the long journey. I felt that I wasn't really geared to that sort of timescale. My Arab guides were certainly on a different timescale from me. They would think basically in terms of a month, and I suspect they thought it was very odd that I became impatient with slow progress, or if I had to stop to buy new camels. They thought nothing of spending two or three days loafing around while they got new camels, while I was wanting to get the camels quickly so that we could get on with the journey.'

Navigation also occupied a lot of Margaret's time, and therefore she was working on an hour scale. 'Interestingly at sea, of course, I was working not only on Greenwich Mean Time but also zone time, because when you're travelling east or west you're either gaining or losing time. There's nothing more ridiculous than having a clock that says twelve o'clock while it's actually six o'clock in the morning by the position of the sun in the sky. So I found it very important to think of my time by the hour. But on the greater scale I found it very easy to lose count of the time weekwise. My longest period between landfalls was in fact a month. I was twenty-eight days going from the Canaries to Antigua, and though I found three weeks bearable the last week was absolute agony. It dragged intolerably, and all I could think of was how to pass those few days as quickly as possible.

Such lone journeys usually make people discover certain things about themselves that they did not know before. Margaret found that there seemed to be no limit to which she could not push herself, which she found incredible. She also came back with reinforced religious beliefs. 'I don't think you can subject yourself to the magnificence of creation, which the sea and the sky certainly are, without becoming deeply aware that there is something beyond yourself – call it God, call it what you will. And I found myself much more committed now to the Christian philosophy as a result of what happened.'

Geoffrey embarked on his journey as what he termed a 'sympathetic agnostic', and his experience hadn't altered that. 'I think that whatever you are comes out rather more emphatically than it normally does, but then you revert to type when you get back and get over it.'

MYTHICAL MUGGERS

Helene Hanff

I got a letter not long ago from a woman in London. 'We hear awful reports of the danger of walking around New York at night', she wrote. 'How do you manage? Do you carry a hat pin?' Two days later I was at Saks Fifth Avenue's information desk when I overheard two Englishmen in front of me express disbelief that Saks didn't carry the item they wanted. They turned away and, wanting to be helpful, I hurried after them.

'Gentlemen,' I said, 'what is it you want to buy?'

One of the men pointed to my shoulder bag. 'The gadget you women carry in your handbags to repel muggers', he said.

I told him I'd never heard of such a gadget.

'Every woman in New York carries one', he replied flatly.

What I answered can be read at the end, when it will make sense. First, let's have a brief geography lesson to define what is, and is not, New York.

New York City is situated on Manhattan Island, a narrow strip twelve miles long by less than two miles wide. But it's surrounded by four other cities, three of them much larger than itself. Back in 1898, for political reasons, the four other cities merged with New York City to create a paper monolith called Greater New York. And because Greater Elsewhere means a string of suburbs around a single city, let me be plain about what constitutes Greater New York.

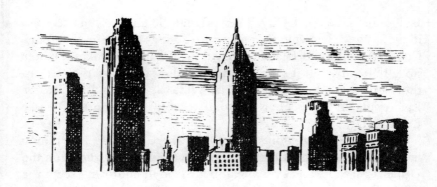

Of the five cities included, the largest is Brooklyn. As many people live in the city of Brooklyn as live in the city of Paris. Next comes Queens, with a population larger than that of Vienna. Add to that the Bronx, with more people than Warsaw; Staten Island, with more people than Cardiff; and New York City, with as many people as live in Greater Liverpool – that is, Liverpool and its suburbs. Like any city, Brooklyn has its well-to-do neighbourhoods and its slums. So does Queens. The Bronx splits into the burnt-out slums of the South Bronx, and the upper-income suburbs of the North Bronx which also has small estates, rolling green acres dotted with palatial homes, and expensive private schools. Ask people in those places where they live, and they'll answer 'Brooklyn', or 'Forest Hills', which is in Queens, or 'Riverdale', in the North Bronx. If they're coming into Manhattan for the day, ask them where they're going and they'll answer: 'To New York.' To them, as to you, New York is the city on Manhattan Island.

Which brings us to crime. Brooklyn, Queens, the Bronx and New York City all have high crime rates. But as the world knows, the USA is a violent country. Every year, a national police report is published listing the cities with the highest per capita crime rates. During the last few years of the seventies, the American city with the highest crime rate was Phoenix, Arizona. In 1980 Miami was first, and Phoenix dropped to second. Greater New York was seventh. Such statistics don't please the news media. How can you get sensational headlines from crime in Phoenix, Arizona? How can you paint a lurid picture, on television, of sunny Miami as the new Babylon? It's much easier to use bad old New York. So the media ignore everyday crime elsewhere, and instead publicize every crime committed in Brooklyn, Queens, the Bronx, Staten

Island and New York City. They present the total to you as 'crime in New York', knowing that *you* will read it as 'crime in New York City on Manhattan Island'. They do it because it makes a better story that way. But it's almost as misleading as if they'd totted up the crime totals for Paris, Vienna, Warsaw, Cardiff and Greater Liverpool, and presented the total to you as 'crime in Greater Liverpool'.

To the lady in London: no, I don't carry a hat pin. Like all my friends, I walk alone at night through every neighbourhood on the Upper East Side, and every neighbourhood in midtown except the Times Square area which is now a slum. I would no more walk alone through a New York slum at night than you would walk alone through a Paris or Liverpool slum at night. And all I could think of to say to the Englishman who informed me that every woman in New York carries an anti-mugging gadget that no woman I know has ever heard of, was: ' You've been reading too many newspapers.'

AUTUMN

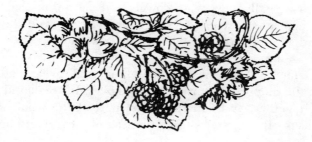

COUNTRY DIARY

Robin Page on the countryside in October

I was looking recently at a nest in an old willow tree surrounded by ivy. It was inhabited by large, wasp-looking things, slightly larger than a queen wasp, and instead of being yellow and black, like a normal wasp, they were yellow and red. They were hornets, and it was quite pleasing to stand and watch them going in and out of their nest, with the ivy in flower, and bees feeding on the ivy as well.

Another odd thing I found was a robin's egg, freshly broken. Quite what a robin was doing at this time of the year laying a fresh clutch of eggs I don't know, but it probably indicates that it has been quite warm despite the rain. Birdsong increases at this time of year, as well – I've noticed for some time robins, hedge-sparrows and skylarks especially. I think it is to do with getting their territory established for next spring, and so they have another burst of melodic activity.

I'm tempted to say, too, that the last of the wild flowers can be seen in November; but this is not strictly true, because if you look hard enough you can always see groundsel or chickweed or some-thing 'on flower'. There were still a lot of flowers out, though – watermint, yarrow, hawkweed and bristly oxtongue, a flower that I particularly like. It's got a yellow flower and the leaves are very bristly; if you've ever been licked by a cow you will know that its tongue is very coarse, much more so than a cat's, and so bristly oxtongue is a perfect name. In my garden I gathered the seeds of my beloved corn cockle. This is a very rare harvest flower, and every autumn I collect the seed. Recently I came across a seedsman who actually sells wild flower seeds; I think that's nice, because it means that people can actually grow wild flowers in their gardens, and won't be tempted to pick them or dig them up from the countryside.

On the land we've been busy ploughing, and it's very satisfying going on the tractor and turning the soil over. It's man and nature working together, and you really feel part of the whole system. As soon as the tractor starts going the seagulls hear it and home in,

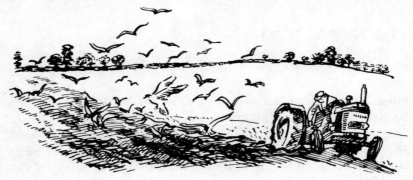

and you're surrounded by flapping wings and birds going down for worms. Hares, too, creep around; they have their ears down and look quite weird, and you can understand why all the folklore about hares started up. Then suddenly they'll spring off, the ears will come up, and they will run away.

At this time of the year I go into a nearby wood because, although people normally associate autumn with dying, it's the time of the fallow deer rut. I look forward to it every year and go at dusk and dawn. Sometimes there are streams of brilliant light and falling leaves, and at other times it's damp and misty and you can hear everything dripping. If you stay very quiet, or hide behind a tree, you hear a groaning noise like a long snore. This is the master buck calling all his lady friends to him, and then small does walk by you very quietly, going to the master. There are also young bucks who are much shyer, who want to get a look into the action but don't often get it, and they will come walking by. I've been within ten yards of a wild fallow deer at this time of the year. It really is a beautiful experience.

Apart from the farming activities and the animal activities there have been human activities too, and I went to a meeting of the Women's Institute which was really quite enjoyable. An old countryman who lives in the village says that WI stands for Women's Interference, and he says that though people say we're run by Parliament, in fact we've been run by the WI for many years! We heard a talk about lacemaking which was most interesting; a lady had brought all different sorts of lace and old bobbins and it was quite fascinating. I am almost tempted to become a member of the WI, if every monthly meeting is as interesting as that one.

The other human activity concerned our neighbouring village, which is Grantchester. The village school is going to be closed, or at least it's threatened with closure, and meetings were held in our village about taking their children. Typically, the education committee are going to increase the size of one school so that they can close another. I think that village schools are part of the fabric of village life and should be maintained at all cost. If a village school closes, part of the village dies, so this is one change in village life that must be resisted as strongly as possible.

A FLEA IN YOUR EAR

There are apparently still about sixty kinds of flea in Britain. A medical expert, some council workmen and the owner of a flea circus give their widely differing views of them

Professor John Maunder, a lecturer at the London School of Hygiene and Tropical Medicine and a flea specialist, was willing to give a demonstration of how fleas suck blood.

'I'm going to put this tube containing fleas upside-down on the back of my hand. The fleas are now on my skin and some of them are interested already – though there's really rather too much light in here for them to be thoroughly happy. . . .'

But they were happy enough to settle down eventually, after they had had a good feel and smell of his skin. John Maunder was demonstrating with the cat flea, the most common of the sixty-odd kinds found in Britain. Central heating and undisturbed fitted carpets are their delight, plus of course a cat.

'The average domestic cat', he said, 'is supporting a colony of something over a thousand adult fleas. There are eggs, larvae, pupae and adults, all of which are *off* the cat except for maybe twenty or thirty which are on the animal at any one time. Fleas are hit-and-run raiders – they jump on to the animal and then jump off. Imagine some lady seeing twenty fleas on her cat. Shock! Horror! She rushes down to the chemist, gets some flea powder, comes back, puts the powder on, and twenty fleas drop off. Great relief. But they're not the *same* twenty fleas that were there originally. For every flea that's on the cat at any one time, a couple of hundred could be waiting their turn to jump on, feed and jump off.'

This enormous community of fleas is distributed around the places where the cat habitually goes, even if it's as infrequently as once a week. They're hit-and-run raiders, and it's the flea's jump which sets him head and shoulders above the rest of the insect world. But it's not because they've got stronger or longer legs – they possess their own unique system.

'They wind up a sort of rubbery spring which they have inside the body. This takes them a tenth of a second. They then release this stored rubbery energy into their back legs and fire themselves off in the air. Every single jump is of exactly the same power, and the flea can only really determine in which direction it takes off and something of the angle of take-off. What is spectacular is that the actual period of acceleration is less than a thousandth of a second. It's the same sort of trick as a boy with a stone and a catapult. He takes a quarter of a second to pull the rubber band back, and then when he releases it the stone flies away in something like a hundredth of a second. It's a way of getting a very much more rapid movement than would otherwise be possible. Were the flea the same size as us, it could jump over St Paul's Cathedral without the slightest difficulty, and could also continue to do so ten thousand times in succession without pausing for breath!'

The fleas on the back of John Maunder's hand were now doing all right. To satisfy their thirst fleas swell to two and a half times their own weight in blood, the equivalent of a sixteen-stone man drinking almost two thousand pints of beer at one sitting! The fleas had now gone dark red, filling themselves up with his blood.

'It's almost a religious experience,' he said. 'It teaches you humility in a way, because you realize that you're not the end of a food chain. We're not predators on all the rest of the world; occasionally some of the rest of the world preys on us.'

The spraying of empty flats for fleas is standard procedure in London Boroughs, and the council workmen have to do a thorough job since the young maggots wriggle their way into the dirt-filled cracks of walls and floorboards. In chrysalis form they can stay there for up to six months and then leap into action at the slightest sign of warmth. Some workmen explained how they go about the task.

'I should think that this flat, that we're going to now, has been empty for about three or four weeks.'

Did they expect many fleas?

'Yes, we always expect fleas. We start spraying before we actually get to the door, in case anything's just inside the door and it comes on to us.'

Of course cat fleas are relatively harmless, but back in the fourteenth century one of its larger relatives, the black rat flea, was the key agent in the spreading of England's worst epidemic, the Black Death. John Maunder took up the subject.

'When the plague arrived in a city, it usually arrived amongst the rats first and it was carried from rat to rat by the rat fleas. Both rats and fleas died of the plague, but the rats died much faster. As the rats gradually died off the fleas, left behind, grew more and more hungry. Finally, in utter desperation, they started to bite man and thus carried the plague from the rat to man. So the appearance of the disease could sometimes be extraordinarily sudden. Something like a third of the population of Constantinople died the very first day they knew they had the plague. This, I think, was why it was so feared.'

The rats themselves had come to Britain via traders from central Asia, and still to this day, in certain areas, the Black Death is endemic among gerbils and marmots. But the black rat fleas had spread the plague almost despite themselves, Professor Maunder explained.

'The plague bacteria can become caught up in spines in the stomach of the flea and eventually completely blocks its gut, so that it cannot feed properly. It always feels hungry, therefore, so instead of feeding just once a day it hops from person to person, desperately trying to feed. Each time it strains and strains, trying to suck some blood in. When it finally decides it can't do so it relaxes, and some of the blood that it's already taken in is regurgitated into the wound, carrying the plague bacteria with it.'

Cat and rat fleas have to be desperate to bite humans – a form of iron rations to them – and if they do, they go for the smooth parts of the body. But the so-called human flea loves to crawl and lodge all round the body, so in the eighteenth and nineteenth centuries it was a common thing to try and catch them with a little device that looked like a hollow cylindrical stick about five inches long. You would unscrew the end of this stick, put some meat inside, screw it together again and put it underneath your pillow. During the night it was much easier for the fleas to crawl in through the holes that were made round the edge of it and get on to the meat than it was for them actually to nip the sleeper. Unfortunately for them, they were a bit too dopey to crawl out again, so in the morning you would go to the fire, undo the end of the stick, pull out the piece of meat with the fleas still attached to it, and drop it on the fire. If you were bothered with fleas in the daytime you put a fresh piece of meat inside, threaded a ribbon through the ring at the top, and wore it hanging round your waist underneath your skirt or down your trouser leg.

Debbie Tomlin was more interested in acquiring fleas than in disposing of them, since she used to run a flea circus.

'We had one riding a little three-wheeled bicycle. We harnessed Percy on to the side-saddle in such a way that he walked on a drum on the back, moving the bicycle. Then we had the chariots, which were more than a hundred times the weight of the flea. We called these fleas Pierre and Pedro and they would have a little race. While they were racing, we put on the duellists. They were harnessed to a stand and facing one another, and in their legs we put a little sword made of cardboard and balsa with handles. Really when they were holding those swords they thought it was something that they could grab hold of to get out of that harness. All the time the swords were going together. Pity they weren't steel, because they would have made a lovely noise.'

These were only some of Debbie's acts, which used props specially made by a jeweller. The fleas worked in a little circus ring about a foot across, and the audience of about fifty a show peered down from tiered benches. Debbie's late husband, Len, had started the circus in 1929. Although he paid a pound a dozen to anyone who would supply him, he always ran short of fleas.

Debbie explained how their landlady at Margate had once tried to help them when they were getting desperate for performers.

'Get your coat on,' the landlady said, 'we're going on the knocker.'

That was a foreign language to Debbie – on the knocker? Anyway, they went up one street and down another. Debbie asked her what she should say.

'Just go up and say, "Madam, I don't know whether I'm at the right house, but we run the performing fleas at Dreamland Park and someone told us that you may have a few fleas available." '

Debbie got chased up the road, insulted and sworn at, but some people did agree to lure their fleas from the wainscoting, and were supplied with rolls of cotton wool, tweezers and an electric fire to do it with. The fleas safely harnessed, the Tomlins would bare their arms and legs to fortify the new performers before they joined the troupe, but their blood had to be pure. If the ring-master had been to the pub just before the show began, the results could be disastrous.

'If you fed the fleas after you'd had a drink, you'd have Percy falling off his cycle, because the liquor goes into your bloodstream and affects the fleas.'

One of the artistes was trained to lie upside-down and juggle with a ball made of balsa wood, and it was this trick that proved the undoing of Jack Woods, a friend of the Tomlins.

'He used to listen to us demonstrating the show,' Debbie said, 'and he thought he could do it. So we let him have a go. Now a flea won't work if it's cold. You either have to touch it and squeeze it very gently with your fingers, or breathe on it. So we said to Jack: "Be careful, it's cold. Either touch him slightly with your fingers or just pick him up and breathe on him gently." "Right", he said.

'Well, the show was going fine. Len and I were outside and getting quite a few people in. All of a sudden Jack came out. "Had an accident!" he said. "I can't talk. . . ." So my husband says, "What's the matter? Got a cold?" "No . . . have to get a drink of water." So I says, "What's the matter, Jack?" "I've just swallowed one of the artistes. I'll have to go to the hospital." Instead of blowing, Jack had sucked, and since it was the juggling flea the piece of balsa wood he was playing with went down his throat too!'

WEAR AND CARE - UPHOLSTERY

Muriel Clark

The first thing to look at is not the covers, but your lifestyle. In a family home with sticky-fingered small children and pets it's wiser to choose upholstered furniture which has wooden arms. It doesn't wear as readily as the kind with upholstered arms, and marks can easily be sponged off the wood.

When it comes to coverings, there are any number to choose from, but again you've got to think about how the furniture is going to be used. Upholstery coverings like tapestry and leather and wool moquette were very popular in my childhood. You can still buy leather and it really is tremendously robust and durable, but you need a fairly fat cheque book.

Wool moquette is also expensive, though less so, and it's considered a little old-fashioned now. And if you've got a cat in the family for goodness sake don't buy this covering, because it's a bobbly material and the cat will simply love sitting up on its hind legs and picking at it. Moquette is rather like carpet, in fact, and you can get both plain and embossed kinds. It is very hard-wearing, and wool is a material which is relatively easy to keep clean.

Dralon velvet is probably the most popular upholstery fabric around today. Though it looks as if it ought to be in my lady's parlour, it really is a surprisingly hard-wearing material, but you do need to be careful not to let it get too soiled.

A lot of the tweeds on chair covers are woven from man-made fibres or at least contain a percentage of man-made fibre, which increases their wearing qualities. If you buy a tweed covering or one of those fashionable soft folkweave ones, do choose one that's closely woven because it will wear very much better.

Then of course there's linen, the cretonne type of printed linen. Again this is usually mixed with a fairly high percentage of nylon or polyester to increase its wearing properties. Some people find it difficult to keep clean if they sit around in dirty clothes, and have animals and children. The best way of dealing with this problem is to have loose covers. I have these on wooden armchairs and they zip off for easy washing. This is another point to note if you're going to have a real family living-room. Look for covers which will zip off because you can have them dry-cleaned or wash them. You might also consider having a spare set, which is both practical and enables you to change the look of your room.

Vinyls are quite a good substitute for leather, but do look for a fabric-backed vinyl, which is the best type. The worst danger with vinyl is tearing, because it can be quite difficult to repair, though you can buy special repair kits so all is not lost if the worst happens. Do beware of getting biro ink or hair oil on it, or any creamy, greasy substance. It's almost impossible to get such a stain off, because you must never use any kind of grease-removing solvent cleaner on vinyl since it just dissolves the material.

As a general rule, the more you pay, the more you get. The wooden-armed chairs are often cheaper than a fully upholstered chair, but of course they aren't quite as comfortable, and aren't very suitable for a draughty room. But they're lighter to move around, which is an important point too.

Now a few words about cleaning and general care. Although you don't actually see it, there's obviously as much dust on furniture whether it's wooden or upholstered, so it's quite a good idea when you're vacuuming the carpet to put the small upholstery nozzle on for five minutes once a week. If you don't, when someone comes in and sits down to watch an exciting television programme you get an eight-, nine- or ten-stone weight on top of all that dust, wriggling about and grinding it all into the upholstery. On fabric upholstery, but not on vinyl or leather, from time to time take a little pad soaked with spirit cleaner and just go over the parts which get extra grubby, such as the arms and the back part where people's heads rest. You'll be surprised at how much soiling comes off.

When it gets more generally soiled you can shampoo your upholstery in exactly the same way as a carpet. You can buy useful little gadgets for doing this – a special head with a tank behind it for holding the upholstery shampoo, which can be the same type as carpet shampoo. Go over the whole piece of furniture with this, but be careful with the overlap areas. You can have it cleaned professionally, too, with a special steam cleaning machine, which makes a super job of it. It costs more, of course, but if you have an expensive suite that's got badly soiled, it's probably worth the money.

CHARLES CAUSLEY

The West Country poet, writer and broadcaster talks about his life and work

I was born a provincial and London was always, and still is, the most magical place in the world for me. I still leap out of the train at Paddington as I did when I was young, quite confident that something marvellous is going to happen before I go home again, and it still does. So it was the most natural thing in the world for me, at the age of fifteen or sixteen, to send my first plays to London and try to get them broadcast by the BBC. They were in fact broadcast not in London but in Bristol, although I did graduate – if that's the word – up the line later on. My home town is Launceston, pronounced Lahnson. It's a town on the border of Cornwall and Devon and I've always felt, although I am indeed a Cornishman, like somebody who lives in a frontier town. My eyes have always been turned east towards London, rather than west towards the Isles of Scilly.

I came to poetry a little later, during the war, when I was serving on a destroyer. One can't write a play or a novel or even a short story on the lower deck of a ship, but I found that I could scrub the deck and peel the spuds and do my job in the radio office as well as write poems in my head, and in a sense I've gone on doing that ever since. It's a much harder discipline than writing prose, and I've tried to stick to my work as a poet for the very fact that I find it difficult: increasingly difficult as time goes by, like breathing.

I didn't have a particularly bookish background. My father was a casualty of the First World War, and I was an only child. I don't remember any poetry in my home at all, and I didn't catch on to it until I was about thirteen or fourteen. But I was always a fanatical reader: I used to read my mother's two-shilling novels, matchbox labels, train tickets – everything. I've always been totally absorbed by reading.

After I'd got a scholarship to the grammar school I came home one day and asked my mother what she thought I should be when I eventually left school, and she said, in all seriousness – I can quite understand why she did – that she thought I should try for a job as a solicitor's clerk. In those strange, class-ridden days this was thought to be a really good job, and about the top as far as I was concerned. Alas, I think I agreed with her. However, I left school at fifteen and got a job first with a builder and then in the office of an electrical company. Then along came Hitler, and the only good deed he ever did in a naughty life, as far as I was concerned, was to extricate me from that boring office with all those nice people and set me down in a ship which I loathed and hated and feared but which totally changed my life, because I began to write poetry.

The Times Literary Supplement once described my poetry as having always been considered suitable for children in the way that nursery rhymes and ballads are, 'for their surfaces, though strange, are accessible, and their rhythms and rhymes strong and encouraging'. This is part of a typical poem called 'Timothy Winters',* which I wrote about a real boy when I was teaching in a primary school.

> Timothy Winters comes to school
>   With eyes as wide as a football pool.
> Ears like bombs and teeth like splinters:
>   A blitz of a boy is Timothy Winters.
>
> His belly is white, his neck is dark,
>   And his hair is an exclamation mark.
> His clothes are enough to scare a crow
>   And through his breeches the blue winds blow.
>
> When teacher talks he won't hear a word,
>   And he shoots down dead the arithmetic-bird,
> He licks the patterns off his plate
>   And he's not even heard of the Welfare State. . . .

Children react differently to that kind of poem from the way that adults do. Though I don't actually write 'children's poetry', because I don't believe in poetry with water, lots of my poems have been taken over by children. The point about writing as far as I'm concerned is communication. You have to leave a space where the reader's imagination can work.

I found that I had a children's audience quite by accident. I remember very clearly going up to our local greengrocer's one Saturday morning about fifteen years ago. I was standing in the queue waiting to buy a lettuce, and two little girls, one aged about six and the other about eight, whom I certainly didn't know, were giving me that old electric blue stare. I knew they were going to say something, that I was going to get something on the chin, and eventually one of them stepped over and said, very politely, 'Excuse me, are you the man who makes the poetry?' It was splendid phrase, a sort of Chinese phrase – 'making something', as one might make a table or a chair. I admitted rather cautiously to being that man, and she turned to her sister. 'Ah, yes,' she said in a very grim tone of voice, 'it's him.' Then they joined hands and recited one of my poems together in the middle of the shop. It was a splendid moment.

The poem was one I'd written to try and express something about night fears, which I found children suffered from a lot. I learned about this when I was teaching young children, or trying to teach them – in fact they were teaching me. I wanted to do something about it, and the result was 'Colonel Fazackerly',** which begins:

> Colonel Fazackerly Butterworth Toast
> Bought an old castle complete with a ghost,
> Someone or other forgot to declare
> To Colonel Fazack that the spectre was there. . . .

Some people might expect a child to enjoy the rhythms of that though not necessarily to understand all the nuances, but I think, on the contrary, that children are subtle and experienced and far-seeing, and pick up clues in poetry. Indeed in all art and all aspects of life they see much more sharply than we adults would care to admit. As a teacher I kept finding that all the time, and to me it was quite frightening. I loved teaching, but I'm not being coy or modest when I say that I know I got more from the children than ever they got from me. They are a strange race of beings who disappear at the age of about fourteen or fifteen and go into another land somewhere or other. The world of childhood is very mysterious.

I originally went into teaching to give myself time to write poetry in the holidays, but it turned out to be a ludicrous decision because I found as time went by that it didn't work like that at all. Notions, ideas – what for want of a better word might be called 'inspiration', though I don't like that word at all – come when one is totally exhausted and relaxed, thinking about something else. Then one gets visited by these thoughts from outside. This used to happen every day when I got home from school with seventy exercise books to correct. But now I'm a full-time writer.

Recently I spent some time in Australia, where I was invited to read at the Adelaide Festival, which was marvellous: a meeting of lots of poets from that area whom I had never met before. Poets are a kind of international gang, and it could be very dangerous to have a squad of twenty or thirty poets! I gave many readings in Australia after that, and found it a delightful experience. While I was in Australia I looked for relics of my great, new-found hero, Ned Kelly. As a border-man myself, I see him as standing on the borders of society and of life. Some time I hope to write something about him.***

*From *Collected Poems 1951–1975* by Charles Causley, published by Macmillan
**From *Figgie Hobbin* by Charles Causley, published by Macmillan
***I did. The poem 'Beechworth' (also the name of the town in New South Wales where Kelly, aged sixteen, received his first gaol sentence) appeared in *The Listener*, 18 June 1981

WOMBLES FOR ADULTS

Elisabeth Beresford, creator of the delightful and popular Wombles of Wimbledon, explains that their appeal is by no means limited to children

I think probably my most unlikely Womble 'experience' occurred when I was asked out to South Africa to open their first-ever book fair. I was only there for about a fortnight, but every single day I was giving about four talks to children in school halls and libraries and all over the place. But the one that really sticks in my mind most clearly was when I was asked to go and talk in a Zulu township.

The person going with me was a very nice Afrikaaner librarian called Michael. We were driven into this very big township and up to a large hall, which was jammed. They reckoned that there were about two thousand Zulus there, of all ages, and there were just the two of us on the platform. Literally as I got to my feet, I realized that I couldn't possibly translate something like the Wombles of Wimbledon into anything relating to the way the Zulus think about life. I decided instantly to turn them into just small, magical people; so, very slowly and carefully, I acted out the stories from the television scipts. The Zulus were a magnificent audience, sitting absolutely still and listening to every word.

After twenty-five minutes I sat down totally exhausted, and it was then that I learned something which I didn't know before: if Zulus like you they don't clap, but give you a high-pitched ululation – a kind of howling noise. Two thousand Zulus doing that is pretty impressive. They also raise their right arm – the spear-throwing arm – and move it backwards and forwards. That's about the nicest accolade they can give you. But you should try standing up there with just one other person, with two thousand Zulus coming slowly towards you giving the Zulu war chant! Michael seized hold of my skirt and said in a sort of strangulated, South African-accented whisper: 'Liza, remember the thin red line and retreat with me, step by step.'

People in many foreign countries do identify with the Wombles and know what they are about. I don't know about behind the Iron Curtain, but I have had one letter from behind the Bamboo Curtain. A cartoon film is being made in America, of which I've seen some little bits. It's terribly funny because all the characters speak in strong American accents. A parcel reached me last year from a student at the University of Grenoble in France, who had written her degree thesis on the Wombles and was sending me a copy of it. She had done what is called a critical path analysis at the back of this enormous thesis, which included among other things the Wombles' social and sex life, about which she knew far more than I did. But it's a very nice tribute to have. Then there was a Japanese professor of English from Tokyo University who came to see me with a whopping great sheaf of papers. He sat down opposite me, polished up his spectacles, then leaned forward and said, very carefully, 'Now tell me, character of Great Uncle Bulgaria is based on that of Dr Johnson. How so?' I thought this couldn't be happening to me, but it was.

Some grown-up people do take it very seriously, but not all. On another occasion that is very fresh in my memory I was asked by the Captain, officers and crew of HMS *Ark Royal* to go down and be their guest and to present them with a large Womble mascot. I was very flattered and thrilled, of course. I went down to Ply-mouth, where the ship was in for a refit, but I didn't really know what it was going to be like on an enormous naval ship. When I was picked up by a lieutenant-commander I was in full evening rig, because it was an evening do. As we got down to the *Ark Royal*, this vast bulk in the darkness, all the sailors were lined up and started to pipe me on board. I suddenly realized that I was going to have to nip up and down ladders, and I was wearing a long skirt. So I turned to the lieutenant-commander and whispered, 'How do you feel about carrying a lady's handbag?' 'No trouble at all, ma'am', he said; he took off his cap, took my handbag, put it inside his cap and then put his cap under his arm. 'The Royal Navy are marvellous!' I thought.

We climbed on board and I was taken up to the Captain's day-room which was full of gold braid. I was the only woman there. They were terribly polite and nice, but it was all a bit starchy. The place was ringed with stewards, also in their number ones. I had forgotten that I was going to present a trophy with what we call a 'Rent-a-Womble', which is a small schoolmaster in a Womble costume. Small because otherwise they look a bit frightening, and schoolmaster because they're used to dealing with children and they know how to cope with crowds. This chap had already arrived on board, unknown to me, and while we were all making very stilted conversation in the Captain's day-room there was a kind of scratching on the bulkhead and a rather nervous voice said: 'Excuse me, sir, somebody to see you.' The Captain said: 'Oh, all right, send him in.'

They drew aside the curtain, and the Captain half got up – at that moment into the day-room stepped Great Uncle Bulgaria . . . life-size. The Captain stopped, frozen, half in and half out of his chair. The whole place went absolutely quiet. Then the Womble got me in his sights, opened up his furry arms and said 'Mother', and the whole thing just collapsed. I'd never seen grown-up sailors weeping with laughter before, but they did that time.

PHOTOGRAPHING ROYALTY

Norman Parkinson has been a professional photographer for some fifty years and has made many studies of the Royal Family. He lives on the island of Tobago in the Caribbean

If you are a photographer, using this wayward machine called the camera, you have to command it and to realize that you're a craftsman. You must get in, behave yourself, take some good snaps, and get out. And if somebody like the Queen Mother, who has only a certain amount of spare time, is prepared to spend some of it with you, you should be on your best behaviour and get some really good pictures.

The picture of the Queen, the Queen Mother and Princess Margaret, all in royal blue capes, that I took for the Queen Mother's eightieth birthday was one that I had proposed several months before. I had a message when I was in New York that there was a possibility of this idea coming off. I felt that it might happen at Windsor, after church one Sunday. So I went to a very smart French fabric agency in New York and bought a half bolt of heavy blue satin which I brought to England with me. I then left it by the TWA check-in desk at the airport, but fortunately my assistant remembered where it was and we ran back and got it! When I landed in England I rang up my friend Hardy Amies and said, 'Do you think that you could make three capes for me?' and he agreed. I suggested three easy capes that could be buttoned up at the back, so that they could be put on over whatever the royal ladies were wearing at the time.

One day in June they turned up after church, all in slightly different garments, looking very attractive. I took some straight-forward pictures first, and then I left the capes in a place where nobody could avoid seeing them. Princess Margaret, who is always a great help on these occasions, said, 'What are these?' I must admit that I had primed her a little in advance. The Queen Mother was delighted with the idea, and since they have the right of veto over any picture that, once printed, they don't like, I suggested that they should try them on. Then of course we had this delightful scene, which could obviously not be photo-graphed, of everybody doing up each other's buttons at the back! If my picture is going to be a piece of history, and perhaps it will become that, it's without fashion. It has a sort of sturdy royal base, and I think that this alone will make it live.

I took another, more formal, picture of the Queen Mother at that time, wearing her tiara and lovely jewels, and looking at me out of a window with raindrops on the pane. I think it is my favourite picture of her alone, because it's quite an impression-istic picture and it captures a lot of the sparkle which she possesses.

It was taken with a very small camera. I was out in the rain and the Queen Mother was saying, as always, 'Come in, Mr Parkinson. You'll get so wet.' But I snapped on, and when I showed her the pictures she was amazed that the miniatures she was wearing of her husband and herself were so clear even through the glass and, as she said, '. . . on such a small camera'.

When I'm photographing the Royal Family it's a job of work for them, so I like to make it as pleasant as I can. I think it's a terrible chore having your photograph taken anyway, although the Queen Mother seems to enjoy it. We take an hour or so, and I pull Polaroids all the time so that they can see how we're getting on – there's a transference of confidence. They can see immediately what I'm doing, and if they don't like it they're the first to say so.

I live now on Tobago, in a house with no telephone, and if people, including royalty, want to contact me they send telegrams. Textel has a little office in town about ten miles away, and a man comes, not with a cleft stick, but on a motorbike. He goes *put put put* ten miles there and ten miles back, and he's already read the telegram anyway. He will say, 'You'll be pleased with this, Mr Parky', or 'This isn't so good, Mr Parky.' And if I'm there he gets his bottle of Guinness and a dollar. We're very good friends.

My other enterprise on the island is sausage-making. I started it because I'm really as much a farmer as I am a photographer, and we couldn't find decent sausages on the island. I've always had farms and I'm very fond of pigs. The sausages are no different from other sausages except that they have meat in them. Sausages are catching on in the USA and I have registered my brand name for America. I hope that the star-spangled banger will be the great export!

CHRISTMAS PUDDING

Two Christmas recipes from Mary Berry, to be made in the autumn to enable them to mature. First, a pudding to serve eight people

2 oz (60 g) self-raising flour
1 coffeespoon mixed spice
12 oz (350 g) mixed dried fruit

3 oz (90 g) fresh white breadcrumbs
3 oz (90 g) shredded suet
1 oz (30 g) almonds
3 oz (90 g) carrot
1 small cooking apple
1 rounded tablespoon chunky marmalade
4 oz (125 g) soft brown sugar
2 eggs, beaten

Grease a 1½-pint (900 ml) pudding basin. Sift together the flour and mixed spice. Put the fruit in a large bowl with the bread-crumbs and suet. Roughly chop the almonds. Peel the carrots and apple, coarsely grate, and add to the bowl with the almonds and

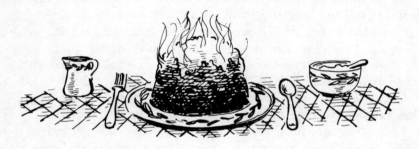

marmalade. Stir in the spiced flour and sugar and mix well together, then stir in the eggs and beat thoroughly. Turn into the basin, cover the top with greaseproof paper and a foil lid, and sim-mer gently for 6 hours. Lift out of the pan, leaving the greaseproof and foil in place. Cool, cover with a fresh foil lid, and store in a cool place until required. Simmer for 3 hours on Christmas Day.

CHRISTMAS CAKE WITH PINEAPPLE

A traditional cake with a difference, this recipe has proved very popular

2 oz (60 g) glacé cherries
7 oz (200 g) self-raising flour
8 oz (250 g) can crushed pineapple
5 oz (150 g) butter

4½ oz (140 g) soft brown sugar
2 large eggs, beaten
2 tablespoons milk
12 oz (350 g) mixed dried fruit

Pre-heat the oven to 325°F (160°C, gas mark 3). Grease an 8 inch (20 cm) round cake tin and line it with greased greaseproof paper. Halve the cherries and roll in flour. Drain the pineapple very thoroughly. Cream the butter and sugar together in a bowl. Beat in the eggs, adding a tablespoon of flour with the last of the egg. Fold in the rest of the flour, the milk and last of all the fruit, including the pineapple and cherries. Bake in the centre of the oven for about 1¾ hours, until pale golden brown and shrinking away from the sides of the tin. Leave to cool in the tin, then remove the paper and store in a plastic container in the refrigerator.

Recipes for almond paste and royal icing are on page 204.

KEYNESIANISM AND MONETARISM

Frances Cairncross was economics correspondent of the Guardian *at the time of this broadcast, and is now editor of its Women's Page*

Monetarism is a term that's bandied about a lot these days, but many people have only a vague idea, if that, of what it means. It's usually contrasted with Keynesianism, so it will perhaps be helpful if I define that first.

Keynesianism takes its name from John Maynard Keynes, who is regarded by most economists as the father of liberal economics in Britain. He was a very distinguished economist who produced most of his writing in the 1920s and 1930s, and some in the early 1940s. Before Keynes, most economists believed very much the same sort of ideas as the present government.

In the period at which Keynes was writing two things had happened in Britain. First of all, in the mid-1920s Winston Churchill decided to fix the exchange rate of the pound in terms of gold at a level which was rather high, much as we have at the moment. Partly as a result of that, Britain in the mid-1920s did not enjoy the boom which a lot of other countries had, and went into rather severe recession.

Keynes made two points about this situation. First of all, he felt that it was very wrong to have such a high exchange rate, and realized that it was an important contributory factor to the recession. The second point, and the one for which he's most widely remembered, is that he suggested a way of dealing with that kind of slump. He noted that one of the problems was that prices were tending to fall, and people were saving an enormous amount of money. In fact I know a lady of sixty who can vividly remember her mother saying to her, before the war, 'Don't buy that now, dear. If you wait a few weeks the price will come down.' Of course everybody did just that; the result was that nobody bought anything, and a severe slump was created. So Keynes suggested that the government should borrow from all those people who were saving such a lot of money, and use this money to pay for projects such as building and repairing roads.

At the time the government didn't like this idea. Governments then tended to believe in the need to balance the budget absolutely, come what may. But as the 1930s went on a lot of countries in effect adopted Keynesian policies because their governments needed to pay for very expensive rearmament programmes. In a way, therefore, it was almost by accident that the sort of policy that Keynes was advocating brought the world out of the slump of the late 1920s and early 1930s.

After the war Keynesianism came to mean something different. Keynes himself had made a prophetic remark about important men of action being the prisoners of some long-dead economist, and a lot of British politicians of the post-war period had their ideas on economic thinking enormously influenced by what they believed Keynes thought. Keynes, if you remember, was talking about a period of very serious recession. Since the war, however, people have tended to regard the cure for periods when unemployment was rather higher than usual as the government spending more money. Keynes didn't in fact talk about what happened if there was inflation, but he was aware that this might be a serious problem in the future.

What we have seen in the last twenty years is a steady and rather horrifying acceleration in the rate of inflation, and because of that, in the last ten years particularly, many economists have started to think more about the need to do something about inflation. Those economists whom people call monetarists have argued that one of the reasons for very rapid inflation has been precisely the government borrowing to finance higher spending which Keynes himself advocated as a cure for recession.

Monetarists are basically economists who are more concerned about inflation than about growth and expansion. The people who are now described as Keynesian are basically economists who are mainly worried about unemployment and about expansion, and regard inflation as a rather secondary problem. I think that's the closest one can come to a definition of the difference between them. Monetarism has now appeared as a brand-new school of economic thought under the Conservative government, but it has in fact been around for a long time. What it says, in a nutshell, is that the rate at which prices go up is fundamentally determined by how much money is circulating in the economy and the rate at which the money supply is increasing. The obvious answer would seem to be not to print any more money, but it's not quite as simple as that. Printed money is a fairly small part of the money supply. If you go into the supermarket you're just as likely to pay for your groceries with a cheque as you are with hard cash, and you might well pay for a pair of shoes with a credit card. There are many more methods of payment than ready money, so really we need to regard money as we would any other commodity, in other words as something that has a price. If there's a glut of tomatoes, for instance, then the price or the value of tomatoes comes down. If there's a glut of money then the value of money goes down.

That's a very simple way of viewing the problem, though, and it has a more complicated side. It's all very well to say that if the money supply doesn't grow, prices will slow down and so therefore will the rate of inflation. When you start asking yourself why it happens, and what the link is by which it happens, then you get into quite muddy water. It has to be thought through along these lines. If there isn't much money around, interest rates are higher, because they are the price you pay to borrow money. If interest rates are high, companies can't afford to borrow enough, so they have to make economies somewhere else. One of those economies is making some of their workers unemployed. The rest of the workforce will be frightened by these redundancies into asking for smaller wage increases. Then, since wages are one of the main factors that go to make up prices, prices won't rise so fast.

Some people wonder if saving money, as opposed to spending it, helps in any way. The answer is that it depends on what you do with the money that you save. We come now to a rather different part of the jungle, as it were, which is the question of what causes the money supply to go up in the first place. Can the government stop the money supply rising? Many economists think that the two factors that determine what happens to the money supply are how much the government borrows, and how much industry borrows. If you save money by, say, buying a National Savings Certificate, the government needs to borrow that little bit less, because in this instance you're lending that money to the government. So if people save like that it does stop the money supply rising so fast. However, if you save by going out and buying a penny black or a valuable antique armchair, it really doesn't help at all because it has no effect on the money supply.

If the present government's monetarist policy works, the result should be low inflation, or no inflation. But of course on the way to the end of the rainbow we are going to experience high unemployment, largely as a result of the policies that the government has adopted in trying to bring inflation down. High unemployment isn't inevitable – if everybody who is at work today decided tomorrow that they were going to accept a much lower living standard, we would have less unemployment, though there would still certainly be some because we're in the middle of a world recession as well. But to some extent unemployment is the inevitable result of a period of very high inflation. What Mrs Thatcher's government wants to do is to bring inflation down. It believes that inflation is a much greater evil than unemployment, while other people think that unemployment is much more dangerous than inflation – it is something you can argue about for hours. But the present government is much more worried about what's happening to prices than about what's happening to jobs.

MYDDLE - PORTRAIT OF A PARISH

David Hey, a lecturer in local history at Sheffield University, has edited Richard Gough's intimate, contemporary account of a Shropshire parish in the late seventeenth century*

Every family was expected to go to church in the seventeenth century and they all had individual, box-shaped pews with little locks which they opened to get into, and fastened again at the end of the service. Richard Gough did something quite remarkable – he took the seating plan of Myddle church and wrote the history of each family in turn, so we have an account of the complete community of Myddle as it was late in the reign of William III.

He was interested above all in human nature, in all the little foibles of his neighbours, which he recalls in the most marvellous and scandalous detail. The best way to illustrate this is by quoting him direct.

Thomas Downton, by his parsimoniouse living, had . . . gott a good stocke of catell, and was in a condition to live well; butt unexpectedly hee married a wife with nothing. Her name is Judith – shee was brought up all her lifetime as a servant in some alehouse or other, and shee proved such a drunken woman as hath scarce beene heard of; shee spent her husband's estate soe fast that it seemed incredible.

. . . my aunt Kathrine . . . was soe extreme fatt, that shee could not goe straite foreward through some of the inward doores in the house, butt did turne her body sidewayes; and yett shee would go up staires and downe againe, and too and fro in the house and yard as nimbly, and tread as light as a girl of 20 or 30 years of age. This, perhaps, to some, may seem idle to speake of; but, indeed, I thought it a very strange thing.

Richard Gough was a yeoman farmer. We know that he lived about a mile away from the church and that his family had lived there, at the hamlet of Newton-on-the-Hill, for about five generations. He was a well-to-do farmer, not quite a gentleman, but obviously a respected man in the parish. We know that he was a well-educated man – he went first to the village school, and eventually became clerk to the most influential justice of the peace in the county; his text is peppered with Latin quotations. In his attitudes he seems to have been very orthodox. He supported the Government and the Church of England, and wrote very much from what we would now call a middle-class point of view.

Gough seems to delight in tales of murder and scandal, but he could also write very generous and shrewd comments about his friends.

Richard [Gittins] the eldest and the 4th of that name, was a good country-scoller, and had a strong and almost miraculous memory. He was a very religiouse person, butt hee was too talkative.

Gittins was a gentleman farmer, one of the wealthiest in the parish, and sat at the very front of the church; however not all the gentlemen in the parish were of quite the same sort of character. Balderton Hall, a building which still survives, is a fine Elizabethan timber-framed house. It changéd hands no less than seven times in just over a hundred years, and the occupants that Richard Gough describes vary from the pious rector of Hodnet to the wicked Michael Chamber.

Butt the worst of this Michael was, that his lewd consorts were such ugly nasty bawds, that they might almost resemble uglinesse itselfe, and such as were the very scorne of the greatest and vilest debauchees of those times, of which, (the more the pity,) there were too many in this parish. Soe prone is humane nature to all vice.

The ordinary farmers sat in the pews immediately behind the gentlemen of the parish. Richard Gough himself was quite near the front. The labourers and cottagers, however, had to sit right against the wall, squashed into the far corner, up against the door. At the time that Gough was writing, a number of immigrants had recently established themselves in the parish – Myddle was still thinly populated, and there was plenty of room for squatters to come in. The last immigrant to arrive at the time that Gough was writing was Evan Jones, who had the only space that was still available, right up by the south door.

The Thirteenth is a small seat att the South dore of Myddle Church. . . . It was made by Evan Jones . . . of some waste planks and boards that were a spare att the uniformeing of the peiws. This Eavan Jones was a Welshman. Hee couald speake neither good Welsh nor English; hee was servant of Mr Gittins of Myddle, and married with one Sarah Foulke who was born in Myddle, and built a lytle hutt upon Myddle Wood near the Clay lake, att the higher end of the towne and incloased a peice out of the Common. This lytle hutt was afterwards burnt, and haveing a collection made in the parish and neighbourhood hee built a pretty good house.

A large number of stories in Richard Gough's history are about courts and prisons, because he was trained in the law and actually served on the grand jury which tried some of the cases. The law was very severe in those days, and you could be hanged for quite trivial offences. For a solid, respectable, Anglican yeoman farmer Gough might seem peculiarly interested in drunkenness and violence, but these were the stories that country folk told each other and no doubt still do. They are also the stories that stick in the mind when you read the book, because they are very entertaining. But we have to remember that they don't all relate to Myddle – some of them are from villages a few miles away, and some of them go back well over a hundred years. On the other hand, some certainly did happen in Myddle, and some occurred in Gough's lifetime.

The last of the Hoddens, save one ... was Thomas Hodden, who married Elizabeth, the daughter of Griffith ap Reece, of Newton. Hee had issue by her ... and soone after dyed, leaveing his wife a young wanton widow, who soone after married with one Onslow, a quiet, peaceable man; but shee soone grew into dislike of him, and was willing to bee shutt of him. There were other women in Myddle, at that time, that were weary of theire husbands, and it was reported that this woman and two more made an agreement to poyson theire husbands all in one night; which (as it is said,) was attempted by them all; butt Onslow onely dyed; the other two escaped very hardly. This wicked act was soon blazed abroad and Elizabeth Onslow fled into Wales, to her father's relations; butt being pursued, shee was found upon a hollyday, danceing on the toppe of an hill amongst a company of young people. Shee was apprehended and brought to Shrewsbury, and there tryed for her life. Her father spared neither purse nor paines to save her; and, as some say, by the assistance of Sir Richard Hussey ... to whom shee had formerly beene a servant, shee escaped the gallows.

At the southern end of the parish is a place called Harmer. All the fields there were originally covered with water because it was a mere, hence the name. Gough tells us that it was drained in the early seventeenth century, and meadows and pastures created; the farmers in Myddle were very much livestock farmers, interested in rearing beef and dairying. The woodland on the other side of the road from the pastures is known as Harmer Heath, and until the early nineteenth century, well after Gough's time, it was common land, for common grazing. It was also the place where the villagers set out a bowling green, and Gough tells a most amusing tale about some of the people who used it.

Thomas Jukes was a bawling, bold, confident person; hee often kept company with his betters, but shewed them noe more respecte than if they had beene his equals or inferiors. Hee was a great bowler, and often bowled with Sir Humphrey Lea att a Bowling Greene on Hare-meare Heath, near the end of the Lea Lane; where hee would make noe more account of Sir Humphrey, than if he had been a plow-boy. Hee would ordinaryly tell him hee lyed, and sometymes throw the bowle att his head, and then they parted in wrath. But within few days, Sir Humphrey would ride to Newton, and take Jukes with him to the bowles; and if they did not fall out, would take him home and make him drunk.

Gough's neighbours probably did not know that he was writing about them. The book was not published in his own lifetime, and I don't think that he intended it to be published. He certainly wasn't writing for posterity, because on several occasions he will say that someone's life is still fresh in people's memory, so that he need not write any more about him. I think he was simply writing for the instruction of his family and friends. Despite his undoubted interest in all the scandalous stories, he does explain that his history of Myddle has a strong moral purpose.

If any man shall blame mee for that I have declared the viciouse lives or actions of theire Ancestors, let him take care to avoid such evil courses, that hee leave not a blemish on his name when hee is dead, and let him know that I have written nothing out of malice. I doubt not but some persons will thinke that many things I have written are alltogaether uselesse; but I do believe that there is nothing herein mentioned which may not by chance att one time or other happen to bee needfull to some person or other; and, therefore I conclude with that of Rev. Mr Herbert [George Herbert, the poet and hymn-writer] –
> 'A skillfull workeman hardly will refuse
> The smallest toole that hee may chance to use.'

The History of Myddle by Richard Gough, edited by David Hey, published by Penguin

ALTERNATIVE MEDICINE

Allen Sharp

I was what I believe the Victorian novelists would have called 'a sickly child'. I suffered principally from what my physicians variously described as 'bronchitis', 'bronchial asthma' or just plain 'asthma', and which the family called 'a bad chest'. I never knew whether these represented different opinions, different diseases, or different names for the same disease – and didn't much care. I refused to allow my disability to prevent me from having a normal childhood – like having mumps and chicken pox and whooping cough. Between colds, I even managed to push in a few quite rare maladies, normally enjoyed only by explorers and missionaries. Because I received a great deal of medical attention, I couldn't help noticing that my medical attendants appeared to die off quicker than I did. I remember concluding that this must have something to do with their being well.

Though the telephone had been invented, no one ever seemed to use it. People did literally 'fetch' the doctor. Since I was the cause of much 'fetching', and since the doctor lived a goodly distance away, my parents did have occasional recourse to what is now called 'alternative medicine'. The alternative medicine was called Mrs Dagleish, and she enjoyed a local reputation for her skills in midwifery, physic, counselling and laying out – in that order. She had a generally muffled appearance and gave the impression of having been knitted rather than conceived. She was much accomplished in the art of 'drawing inflammation'. She drew my inflammations in all sorts of directions – to my feet with hot mustard baths, to my head with hot potions, and to intermediate parts of my body with poultices. I formed the theory that these were not so much to cure the disease as confuse it, and took some comfort in the fact that I had missed out on blood-letting by several decades. So far as my bad chest was concerned, much value was placed upon the need 'to keep the tubes lubricated'. The lubrication was a mixture of linseed oil and turpentine applied liberally to the throat and chest. It kept flies away in the summer and was almost equally effective with people.

Though I could not recommend many of the family's dietary remedies – boiled onions for colds and red herrings for biliousness, not to mention the prophylactic value of good 'stomach liners' like porridge and steamed suet puddings – there were some things that I positively enjoyed. If, like me, you enjoy being cosseted, there is no better way of cosseting than with preparations such as treacle posset, mint tea or calves-foot jelly. Indeed, I think it was the disappearance of these special delicacies which caused me to give up being ill, since the only advantage of being ill is the pleasure of getting better. It's one thing to curl up in a warm bed with a good book and a treacle posset. It's just not the same with nothing but a multivitamin pill and a cough bottle that isn't even brown and boasts about being decongestant, antispasmodic and expectorant – when all you've got is a bad cough!

A LITTLE LEARNING

Len Tutt is a headmaster who was born in Wales

The Renaissance was about five hundred years late in reaching the valley. It could have missed us completely had it not been for the circulation wars waged between the great newspaper combines in the late twenties and early thirties. Left to our own devices we were *Daily Herald* readers to a man, with the jet setters taking the *News of the World* for Sabbath titillation. Then one morning groups of hungry-looking students came, banging on our doors and flourishing fistfuls of forms in our faces. If only we would agree to sign up to take a different newspaper for six weeks they would get twopence a form and we would be given free, gratis and for nothing a volume of startling thickness, bound in imitation calf and with pages edged in imitation gilt. Most of us licked our indelible pencils and signed on the dotted line.

In a week or so the parcels started to arrive. The book was called *Be Your Own Lawyer*, and words and phrases like 'onus of proof', 'aggregation' and 'estopel' came leaping out of the pages to grab us by the throat. Truth to tell, there was no story line at all, and the books were soon consigned to the front parlour for visitors to see.

Some of the contents did rub off on the more persistent readers, though. Men who had happily cultivated adjoining allotments all their lives started to talk darkly about consulting deeds to establish boundary limits. Mrs Rhiannon Mafeking Hughes threatened to take her neighbour, Fat Martha, to the highest court in the land, complaining that every time Martha hung out her voluminous butcher blue winceyette bloomers to dry they interfered with Rhiannon's ancient lights. She claimed that on a poor drying day she had to have the gas on in her back kitchen from morning to night. Just when things were getting really nasty we were saved by a fresh invasion of students, begging us to make another change in our reading habits. And this time, to our eternal joy and delight, we were to be rewarded with copies of *Be Your Own Physician*.

Now if we knew anything at all about anything at all it was about the human body and all its frailty. We were a community that accepted ill health as the norm, and the surgery was as much part of our social life as the pub and the chapel. We devoured our copies from first page to last and then felt willing, nay eager, to play a full part in the diagnostic process. The road to the surgery became a Via Dolorosa of the halt and the lame, each one carrying a copy of *Be Your Own Physician* with relevant passages marked with strips torn from an old newspaper. Most also carried specimens in medicine bottles – this was standard practice, whether you were going sick with a sprained ankle or to have a boil lanced. The surgery became more like the reading-room at the Institute, alive with the rustle of turning pages and the monotonous rumble of the slow readers building up the more difficult words. When the doctor called 'Next' you went in ready for him, book in hand. 'It says here, doctor, that I've got beri beri. I've tried a couple of Aspros but they don't seem to shift it.'

The surgery was a makeshift affair of corrugated iron, and those in the waiting-room could hear everything that passed between doctor and patient. The fast readers leafed through their books, ready to give a second opinion if invited. There was one occasion when Bron Petti Sing Price, diva of our local amateur operatic society, fooled everyone completely. Her symptoms as she listed them just did not tie up with her diagnosis of laryngitis. The doctor and those in the waiting-room were equally at a loss. Then Dai Dando gave a great shout and burst into the consulting-room, book open to prove his point. 'Bron, you daft ha'porth, you've turned over two pages together. That's what she's done, doctor!'

Goodness knows where it would all have ended had the Medical Aid Committee not acted fast. They moved the surgery to a new venue at the top of a steep asphalt path worn as smooth as glass and which would have tested a sherpa to destruction. Not many people could make it to the top, and the nights were full of muttered curses and the sound of breaking specimen bottles as the sick slipped back down the path with their boot studs striking sparks as they sought to keep their feet. Overnight we were reduced to a situation where only the supremely fit could report sick.

But we were not too worried. We had had another visitation of students and had changed our daily newspaper a third time. This time we all received copies of *Be Your Own Gardener*, and we were too busy cleaning our back gardens of rusting tin baths, old bed frames and collapsed pigeon cotes to be over-concerned about our health for a while.

SUFFER LITTLE CHILDREN

Len Tutt on the agonies and indignities inflicted by the old-fashioned schoolmistress

It is surely ridiculous – but still a fact – that I am haunted by two maiden ladies who terrorized my early schooldays to such an extent that I am reluctant to repeat their names. They were so alike in appearance that they could have been twins, and I never did work out which one was the headmistress and which the assistant. They dressed alike, in corded serge and bombazine, and wore immensely high choker collars of net stiffened with whale-bone. I will never, never forgive Penry Owen for telling me that when the two ladies removed their collars at night there was nothing to support their heads, so they lolled on their shoulders like loosely tethered balloons – I frequently woke up screaming, having seen those awful heads floating about in my dreams. The only discernible difference between them was in their teaching methods. One favoured a flat, heavy-handed slap about the ears, while the other had perfected a straight, two-fingered jab which could shatter oar planks. It was my daily dilemma that, not being able to tell them apart, I was never sure whether to protect my ribs or my ears when they spoke to me.

Their educational philosophy could not have been simpler. Get them young and treat them rough. We were admitted to the school practically straight from our mothers' breasts at three years old, and any child who wasn't well on the way to being literate and numerate by three and a half was a wilful and disobedient child

170

who deserved all that they could inflict on him.

My start was a bad one. My mother had been a teacher herself before her marriage and she'd taught me the rudiments of phonics. For this untoward presumption on her part the 'misses' were determined to cut me down to size. I was hardly in the place before I was lifted on top of a high table and commanded: 'Read that!' Almost out of my wits with fear, I failed to recognize the very first word, 'the'; and, as I had been taught, I tried to build it up phonically – an impossible task. 'Tuh-huh-eh', I tried. It didn't make much sense, but not a lot of things do to a frightened three-year-old, so, anxious to please, I gave it another go. However I had failed to notice that I now had an attendant harpy on either side of me. 'Tuh', I tried, and got a dig in the ribs which left me gasping. 'Huh', I ventured through incipient tears, and got a crack across the head which left my senses reeling. 'Eh', I almost shouted in fear and desperation, and got both a slap and a dig in my already bruised ribs. The class were invited to witness my discomfiture and I was forced to continue. Blinded with tears, I was unable to recognize such old friends as 'cat' and 'sat' and 'mat'. As I was roughly restored to floor level, I heard one hiss to the other: 'So much for madam, with her airs and graces.'

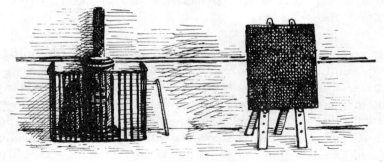

It was assumed that we should be continent from the word go, and no one asked twice whether they might go to the toilets across the playground during lesson time. But accidents were still frequent. The unlucky victim always tried to pretend that nothing had gone wrong, but it was not the sort of situation which one could hide for very long. Suddenly, in mid-sentence, there would be a shriek and we would be showered with globules of venomous spit. 'Someone's been a dirty, filthy beast!' The offender was cuffed and hustled out of his trousers and soundly smacked. But there was worse to come. To send him decently home through the streets he was wrapped, sarong-like, in the school's Union Jack, his trousers rolled and tucked under his arm, for all the world to see his disgrace. It must have been a long walk, tripping and struggling to stay upright in the red, white and blue cocoon.

The other day I was shown a faded photograph of our class, forever frozen at the age of three and a half. The little group is watchdogged by two elderly spinsters. They look harmless enough, and I thought for a moment that I might have been too hard on them. Then I looked more closely. Not one of us is looking out for the birdie. We have got our wary eyes on the two teachers. One liittle girl appears to be near to tears, and is nursing her ribs. There is one good thing, however. In the background the Union Jack is fluttering from the flagpole, so, on that morning at least, no one had been a dirty, filthy beast.

A GIRL AT ETON

Joanna Bentley describes the social and cultural transition from girls' grammar school in Lancashire to this formerly all-male bastion of traditional British education

The very first day I just wanted to go home and cry. I sat in the Chapel on the first assembly and I couldn't believe it – there was just me, and lots of boys. My year were all wearing the uniform that they had worn together over the past five years, and they knew the teachers, and they looked at me and said, 'Oh, that's the girl, *the* girl.' They all regarded me with awe, but nobody really wanted to get to know me properly for the first few weeks. They only wanted to be acquainted with me, so that other people would know that they were acquainted with 'The Girl'. I therefore had no friends at first, so I just absorbed myself in the work, which is no fun if that's all your school life consists of. They were kind to me, though – I think they felt very fatherly. A lot of them thought that I would need looking after, and were willing to invite me for tea, and things like that. But after a few weeks I started to make some proper, deep friendships with people who really wanted to know me, and after that it was just like being at a girls' school.

I come from a vicarage in an industrial town in the north, and I was very much aware of the differences in our home backgrounds, because it really affects the way they treat you. The boys in the north didn't know how to make you feel like a girl – they wouldn't dream of opening doors for you, for instance. The boys at Eton are on the whole real gentlemen, and try to treat me differently. A lot of them are very smooth-talking, but I think that is a cover-up. They've been brought up to be able to smooth-talk – it's part of their way of life, to know the right things to say; but when you get past that they're just like me, and like all the northern boys. All boys have the same kind of feelings, but the boys at Eton know to talk formally at first.

It is a school with all sorts of rules and traditions that don't exist in any other academic environment, certainly not in newer schools. I feel that the uniform itself is old-fashioned, but still necessary, because tradition is very important. I would never condemn the way that the Head Master and the authorities make the boys continue to wear this strange uniform of tails and waist-coat and bow tie. It really does look bizarre to the normal shopper walking through Eton, and yet I think it's such a good idea – it must be carried on because it makes Eton Eton. It's meant to be a place where they breed good Christian gentlemen; it doesn't manage that at all, since they don't go out as good Christian gentlemen, but the traditions contribute towards it, and I think that's great. In fact a few years ago the boys had a poll to decide whether they wanted to wear this uniform or suits, and the result was that more wanted to wear the traditional uniform that they are still wearing now. Perhaps they just didn't fancy the three-piece suits.

I'm very lucky really, because on my list of rules that was prepared specially for girls it says 'Dress – sober', which I take to mean cords and skirts and so on. I do try to conform to what the boys aren't allowed to wear in their spare time and in between lessons – no denims, for instance, or pumps. Usually I wear cords because they are comfortable, and no boys ever criticize them; they never say, 'It's not fair, you can just dress freely. We've got to wear these stupid tails.' I know they just accept it.

It would be impossible for a girl or even a boy to come to Eton in the sixth year, as I did, and absorb themselves and know what was going on straightaway. I needed lots of help – the main thing was the language, which is so completely different from anything I've ever known. They would never use the word 'teacher' here, for example; they say 'beak', which I found really strange. When somebody said to me, 'Which beak are you up to this half?' I just nodded and smiled; in fact it means which teacher is going to teach you this coming half – half meaning term. 'Mess' means to get together and have a good time: 'sock' means food, and if you want somebody to invite you for tea you say, 'Will you sock me?'; 'divs' means lessons, or it could refer to a group of you in the lesson. Those are the main words in Eton's private language. At the other end of the scale, I still have an Oldham accent, which some of the boys make fun of and mimic. It's particularly notice-able because there aren't any other northerners at Eton.

This may sound silly, but I think that Etonians are better-looking than other boys, say Oldham ones. Perhaps it's because their parents can afford things like teeth-straightening and nice clothes and good hairstyles, but a lot of them are really handsome. I don't find it a distraction, though, because I made sure that it wouldn't be. I told myself I wasn't going to try and make boy-friends out of these boys. Although I was going to a boys' school I was going to treat it like a girls' school, or else I wouldn't succeed academically.

If I was in the sixth form in Oldham, the work would be pretty much the same as at Eton, but the teaching would not be so good. They have some really good teachers down here, and the classes are very intensive because they're so small. It's a school of the elite, and I notice it when I'm working with them. Some of the boys are thick, as at normal schools, but a lot of them are sharp and intelligent, which is great because it makes me work and keeps me up to scratch.

WHAT WE SAY - AND THE RESPONSE WE GET

*Professor Randolph Quirk, Vice-Chancellor of the University of London,
and formerly Quain Professor of English Language and Literature,
explains that the way we express ourselves is governed by the kind of
response we hope to receive*

Talking to close friends or members of the family is of course the
easiest thing in the world. At any rate it never occurs to us to
worry about our pronunciation or our grammar, and if we can't
think of the right word, we say: 'Oh, you know – the thingummy,
the what d'you call it', without the slightest embarrassment. But
there's still one respect in which, if we're the slightest bit sensitive
and tactful, we carefully monitor everything we say or hear (for
even family and friends can be touchy) – and that is *response*. In
other words, we don't mind saying something wrongly, but we do
mind about saying the wrong thing.

Every time we say to a child: 'That sounds a bit rude, darling',
we're concerned to pass on this message: your language must not
merely get your meaning across, but it's also got to hit the right
tone and get the right response. We don't have to make this distinction consciously, because the two things are really bound up
together: we simply don't put our meaning across if we've spoiled
the chance of getting the right response.

There seems to be a quite natural and logical grading in our
language-teaching to the next generation. The clamouring two-
year-old says: 'Mummy – dory.' Mummy understands this as a
request – an order, you might say – to tell a *story*. But although she
understands, she'll say mildly, '*Story*, darling', before settling down
to obey. She is beginning the process of ensuring that the young-
ster will be understood by the rest of us who might not be so quick
to realize that 'dory' means 'story'. Later, when as a three-year-old
she says, 'Mummy, tell a story', her mother will reply, '*Please*,
darling', not because *she* needs the courteous extra, but because
she knows it's important if the right response is to come as readily
from others.

But the problem of response gets much tougher when we have
to talk or write to people outside our immediate circle. It's then
that we find ourselves inclined to worry about pronunciation,

grammar and choice of words – again, not so much to get our meaning across, as to get the right response. The commonest and most striking example for many people is the way in which our language changes in church – especially in prayer. I have heard northerners who normally say 'a council grant' so as to rhyme with *pant*, use the vowel we have in *car* or *ah* when they say or sing the words 'Grant us thy peace.' And we are inclined to affect language that is not natural to us when we're speaking to people whom we regard as VIPs.

Just recently, there was a curious instance of this happening in reverse when I was interviewing a young man for a job. He was a northerner, and at one point, when he had to refer to a relative of his, I was surprised to hear him say 'my aunt' with the *ah* sound. He then hesitated and said 'my *ant*'. This was clearly a response problem, and, although I can't be sure what was going on in his mind, I think it was something like this. 'I'm talking to elderly VIPs, so I'd better move outside my own dialect. No: I'd better not – they'll think I'm affected.' So he switched back from 'my arnt' to 'my ant', and I for one thought the better of him – though I'd have liked it still more if he'd had the self-confidence to say 'my ant' in the first place!

Grammatical 'correctness' versus response is another interesting linguistic hump. You know the sort of thing: should we say 'who' or 'whom'? 'Each of us is' or 'each of us are'? 'Taller than her' or 'taller than she'? Is it wrong to begin a remark with 'hopefully' or 'between you and I'? And if you're asked 'Who is it that wants a taxi?', what's the difference whether you reply 'Me and Bob' or 'Bob and me' or 'Bob and I'?

These things are usually treated in terms of correctness: one of the choices ('Bob and I') is right, the others are wrong, and there's nothing more to say on the matter. If the position were as simple and straightforward as that, we'd have a very strange situation indeed – because, of course, a lot of people (including people who don't like the expression 'a lot of people') undoubtedly do say 'between you and I' and 'taller than her'. There are people who believe that 'me and Bob' is wrong and that 'Bob and I' is right – and yet they choose to say 'me and Bob' from time to time. Why? If some expressions are correct and people know them to be so, why shouldn't the same people use them all the time?

It must be obvious, on the briefest introspection, that it is very rare for any of us to wonder – still less to worry – which is actually correct when we hesitate between one expression and another. We don't ask ourselves 'Which is right?' nearly as often as we ask ourselves 'Which sounds better?' Now these aren't just variants of the same question – 'Which sounds better?' doesn't mean 'Which sounds as if it's better English?' What we mean is, 'Which will our hearer or reader *prefer*?' 'Which will have a better *effect* on this particular occasion?' In other words, we are back once again to the idea of response. It is much more important to worry about whether 'taller than her' will sound a bit too breezy or even sloppy to the person we're addressing, or whether – the opposite risk – 'taller than she' will sound priggish and school-marmy. When Shakespeare has his Cleopatra grill the messenger about Antony's wife, Octavia, he puts into her mouth the words: 'Is she as tall as me?' And that helps to transform Cleopatra from being the mighty Queen of Egypt, bringing her down to the level of ordinary people: she becomes just a woman, anxiously comparing herself to a feared rival for her lover's regard.

Not long ago, I read the following remark by a solemn political commentator: 'Enhanced levels of sickness benefits militate in favour of increased absenteeism.' I understood it well enough – especially after I'd translated it to myself as 'If you pay people too much when they're sick, you encourage them to stay off work.' I understood it all right, but my first response was: 'Why does this chap have to write so pompously?' Why, especially when so many of us react in precisely this way? Here is another example: 'The satiated operative is inclined to be non-purposive', which seems to mean 'Once a worker has got all he wants, he stops being ambitious.' Since the translations are surely easier to understand, we can assume that they would also have been easier to write in the first place. So – to reverse the old joke – why be absolutely impossible when with far less effort you needn't even be difficult?

Beauty, as we all know, is in the eyes of the beholder, and so it is with language. What one person hopes will sound friendly and informal will strike another person as sloppy and careless; to avoid giving that impression, we may try to sound precise, elegant, and dignified with an expression that unfortunately strikes another person as stuffy, obscure, and pompous. Misjudging the response in either direction is unfortunate, of course. But thanks to the increased informality in our society and the concerted attack over many years on jargon and officialese, most of us tend to err on the side of seeming careless and even slangy rather than run the opposite risk of sounding uppity and pompous. All the same, the temptations are still there – when we're trying to word an invitation, a notice at the tennis club, or a press announcement of a daughter's wedding: 'After the nuptial ceremony, at which the Reverend John Smith officiated, the gracefully attired bridal party proceeded to a reception at the nearby residence of the bride's father.' Ugh! Sometimes, though, we are right to yield to the temptation. Anything of a legal or regulatory nature has to be in precise legal jargon because the informal translation could be manipulated by the cheats of this world. And there are occasions – for example, in discussing death, or serious illness, or intimate personal problems – when a dignified and formal style is right, even at the risk of being thought pedantic and pompous. A journalist inquiring about the circumstances of a death would obviously be ill-advised to say on the phone: 'Hi, Mr Jones, I'm ringing for a bit of info on just how your sister came to snuff it.'

Response goes right to the heart of the language around us: it's the property of language that most concerns us. And this is true whether we think of response as being our inward reaction to what we hear or read, or whether it is the verbal response we actually make when something is said to us – quickly sizing up the likely response our words will have in their turn.

DR JOHNSON'S DICTIONARY

Philip Howard, Literary Editor of The Times, *on what is arguably the most famous dictionary of the English language**

Dr Johnson's is certainly not the earliest, nor the biggest, nor the most accurate dictionary. It's no use as a dictionary at all nowadays, but in many ways it's the greatest ever written because it was by a first-ranking literary figure. As literature, as bedside reading, and for jokes, it is certainly the greatest dictionary ever compiled.

It's immensely subjective in many ways. It has great flaws in it, and makes astonishing mistakes. Johnson committed an amazing howler under the letter H, for instance, when he said that it:

'. . . seldom, perhaps never, begins any but the first syllable, in which it is always sounded with a full breath except in heir, herb, hostler, honour, humble, honest, humour and their derivatives'. John Wilkes, who reviewed it in the *Public Advertiser*, wrote: 'The author of this remark must be a man of quick appreHension and compreHensive genius but I can never forgive his unHandsome beHaviour to the poor knightHood, priestHood . . .' and so on. Johnson, who was never a man to let the opposition have the last word, got his own back in the next edition. He put a note in under H, reading: 'H sometimes begins the middle or final syllables in words compounded, as "blockhead".'

I definitely wouldn't have thought of him as an obvious lexicographer. One of the things we forget about Johnson is that we know him mainly through Boswell's biography, the greatest in the English language. Boswell, a first-rate first-hand reporter, wrote about Johnson only from the time he got to know him, when Johnson was already the Great Old Man of Literature. We forget about Johnson's desperate, struggling early years when he was a wretched Fleet Street hack, working very hard to make a living, being arrested for debt, and very near collapse for much of the time. He took on the dictionary partly because the idea amused him, but also because he needed the money.

In his own life he was the most undisciplined of men. All journalists have deadline problems, but Johnson had them to such a pronounced degree that they became almost a mania. He could not get down to a piece until after the deadline. He would put it off and put it off; eventually the printer would send round a messenger boy to collect his copy, but he would find Johnson in a room full of people – usually a lot of women, whose company he enjoyed – drinking tea and talking. When Johnson could not escape any more, and it was almost too late to write the piece, he would sit down in the middle of the hubbub and write out those perfect classical periods on his knee.

Dr Johnson's was the first dictionary to use quotations, and one of its important features is that every definition is illustrated with examples from English literature. A biography of Robert Browning said that he educated himself by reading through Johnson's dictionary two or three times, and I sometimes think that Browning's work rather shows it. In his preface Johnson says that he is going to illustrate his definitions of words by reference to the masters of English literature such as Shakespeare, Milton and Hobbes, and that he is not going to use contemporaries except when some particular excellence excites his admiration, because it would be invidious and because history hasn't made up its mind yet which of his contemporaries are good writers and which not. In fact when he gets down to it he uses quotations from his own work considerably, and in one instance at least there's a couplet from Pope which he attributes to himself. If you read Johnson's dictionary – though it's not a book you read from cover to cover but rather one you keep by your bed and dip into – by the time you've finished it you will have read a great part of Shakespeare and a great part of Milton and a great part of Hobbes. You will also have read a great deal of Johnson.

Another criticism of it is that some of the definitions are ludicrously sesquipedalian – that's the sort of word he would use, and what it means is that some of them are far too simple. He defines 'butter', for instance, as an unctuous substance, which isn't really sufficient; and 'parsnip' he defines merely as a plant.

By concentrating so far on Johnson's prejudices and slips I may have unintentionally made the dictionary sound full of mistakes. It isn't, but what comes over strongly is that it is a very human book. I think it's the only dictionary that finds its way into dictionaries of quotations for jokes. One of the famous ones is his definition of 'network': 'anything reticulated or decussated at equal distances with interstices between the intersections'. That is a marvellous piece of Johnsonian grandiloquence. It's also quite a good definition, and lexicographers still admire it. A less well-known one, perhaps, is his definition of 'cough', which most people find amusing: 'a convulsion of the lungs, vellicated by some sharp serosity. It is pronounced COFF.'

Simple words tend to be the most difficult ones to define. A word like 'a', for example, is almost beyond definition, and 'the' or 'table' are quite difficult. When you get to complicated words, something like 'decussated' is very easy to define. Johnson does get some of his definitions wrong, though. There's a well-known story about a woman who asked him why he defined 'pastern' as a horse's knee; he replied: 'Ignorance, madam, pure ignorance.'

Among the dictionary's good points are its huge size, and the fact that most of the definitions are extraordinarily good, while many of them are funny and clever. Some of them are outrageously biased, and he has a terrible go at his enemies. He fought a savage war with Bolingbroke, for instance, and his hatred of him intruded into the definitions. If you look up 'irony' Johnson defines it as 'a mode of speech in which meaning is contrary to the words, as "Bolingbroke was a holy man".' I can't see any other dictionary in the world doing that – it's like somebody attacking Auberon Waugh or Michael Foot in a dictionary.

The other important point about it is the actual scheme of giving the word and then making an attempt at its etymology; some of his etymologies are grotesquely wrong but very funny. Shortly after publication a young Irishman came into the room where Sheridan and others were standing. Johnson was at the window and didn't see him. The young Irishman went over to look at the two large folios on the table – Johnson's dictionary. He opened it at 'helter skelter', and Johnson's etymology said that it was from Old English and Anglo-Saxon, meaning the darkness of Hell. The young Irishman was not convinced and shouted out: 'That's a very far-fetched etymology.' Everyone was appalled, because Johnson was there, and one of them said: 'Well, young sir, I suppose you can give us a better definition, can you?' At once the Irishman said: 'Oh yes, it's the Latin *hilariter celeriter* – merrily and swiftly. Won't that do?' It's a marvellous etymology – but also quite wrong, mind you. They were both quite wrong!

It's foolish to wish one lived in different times from one's own, but I've often thought it wouldn't be a bad thing to have lived in Fleet Street when Johnson was around.

*A new edition, *Johnson's Dictionary: A Modern Selection*, has recently been published by Gollancz

WORDS FAIL ME

Philip Howard talks about his recent book, a compilation of his articles on language that have appeared in* The Times

In an immensely boring union meeting I was once attending somebody said 'across the board', and I started thinking about what that meant. I assumed it must be a table at which people were sitting. Then I looked it up, and found that in fact it's a betting term from the United States. If you want to bet on any of the first three horses in the race you lay your bet 'across the board'. It seems astonishing that it's come to mean what it has, and that when we rant on about 'settlements across the board' what we're actually referring to is Harry the Horse and punters.

The language of politics, another subject that I talk about, has always been slightly devious – it's rhetoric. If you go back to its beginning, to Aristophanes, you will find that Cleon and others used language in a very slippery way indeed and Aristophanes rebuked them for it. Euphemism is one of the tools of the politician's trade, and it's not new. 'Pacification' was a term used in the Vietnam war, when what they actually meant was blotting out everything that moved. But people have been doing that for two thousand years. There's an example in Tacitus, when a British chieftain called Calgacus describes what the Romans do: *'Ubi solitudinem faciunt, pacem appellant'* – 'They make it a place of desolation, and they call it pacification.' So that particular euphemism has been around for a very long time indeed. Churchill could use language in quite a shifty way, and he knew it. There's a marvellous quote from him acknowledging the way that politicians use language: 'How infinite is the debt owed to metaphor by politicians who want to speak strongly but are not sure what they are going to say.'

Among the metaphors of everyday language are grinning Cheshire cats and crying crocodiles. I had always thought that the Cheshire cat was invented by Lewis Carroll, but in fact it came into the language about a hundred years before him. Quite why they are supposed to grin I do not know, though there are about a dozen possible explanations, none of them particularly persuasive. One of them says it smiles because it comes from a County Palatine – it's a snobbish cat; another relates it to a torturer who came from Cheshire and grinned horribly when he was dealing with his victims. 'Crocodile tears' is quite a useful cliché/euphemism – a nice image, an immortal image. Spenser, Shakespeare, Milton, everyone's used it, but whoever first had this strange idea that crocodiles wept hypocritically while they ate their victims? When European civilization first came across crocodiles it wasn't there. Our first record of crocodiles is in Herodotus, who was an immensely curious investigative reporter – if the story had been around then he would certainly have noted it. It can't be dated exactly, but it seems to have come in around the fourth or fifth century AD, when some monks produced a bestiary which had pictures of strange animals with funny stories containing a moral.

Going on to something rather different, Pidgin English is a rich new source of language, and perhaps I should first explain exactly what it is. I think the best definition of Pidgin is an artificial language created when two different languages meet, and the speakers of neither language know the other's language. It comes from business English, from when the Chinese first met British traders. People used to look down on Pidgin as a second-class language, but in some cases it becomes the mother tongue of a community, when it is called a Creole.

Excelsior is a marvellous stuffed owl of a poem by Longfellow, which all schoolchildren used to learn. Just for fun I've translated a couple of verses into Pidgin:

The shades of night were falling fast,	*That nighty time begin chop-chop,*
As through an Alpine village passed	*One young man walkee – no can stop,*
A youth, who bore, 'mid snow and ice,	*Maskee now, maskee ice,*
A banner with the strange device,	*He cally flag with chop so nice,*
Excelsior!	*Topside morefar!*
A traveller, by the faithful hound,	*That young man die, one large dog see,*
Half-buried in the snow was found,	*Too muchee bobbely findee he,*
Still grasping in his hands of ice	*He hand blong colo – all same ice,*
That banner with the strange device,	*Hab got he flag with chop so nice,*
Excelsior!	*Topside morefar!*

Words Fail Me, published by Hamish Hamilton

ANTHONY BURGESS

The multi-talented novelist talks about his life, work and other interests

A number of years ago I wrote a twenty-one chapter novel called *A Clockwork Orange* for Britain, and when I sold it to America it came out as twenty chapters. In the British edition, this story of a young thug who commits all possible crimes ends up with him seeing the futility of violence, wanting to grow up and become the father of a child, a faithful husband and a decent working man. In

England this was regarded as reasonable because people do change, even young thugs. In America, however, they wanted to end on an unregenerate note, with the young thug deciding to be a young thug for ever, and it was out of this version that the film was made. But when the film was seen in parts of the world other than America everybody asked the same question: 'What happened to the last part of the story?' The director, Stanley Kubrick, didn't even know the last part of the story existed. This is unique, because the book has the same title and the same author, and yet it's really two different books. I'll never allow this to happen again – I only allowed it to happen then because the Americans said they wouldn't publish it unless I cut out the last chapter. I needed the money, so I said they could go ahead. Never again.

The book was written in rather strange circumstances, admittedly – I wrote five novels that year because I thought I was dying. I came back from the Far East, from Borneo, with a suspected cerebral tumour, and entered the Neurological Institute in Bloomsbury where I underwent all kinds of painful tests. I wrote a novel about that, too. . . . At the end they said, 'We can't do much about it, but you still obviously have the symptoms of a cerebral tumour, so we'll send you home.' They gave me a year to live, which I didn't know about although my wife did. She tried to keep it to herself but eventually told me.

When I heard this I didn't quite believe it. I didn't feel in the least depressed, and I thought the only thing to do was to get down to some writing before it was too late. So I wrote my five and a half novels in that year and gained the reputation of being too hard a worker. In Britain novel writing became a gentlemanly activity with E. M. Forster, who only wrote five novels. That was regarded as enough for any gentleman to write in a lifetime, and I was writing five novels in a year – this was very ungentlemanly. I'm told it's depressing for anyone who wants to write a thesis about my work, and there have been, God help me, theses written about my work – mostly in America. But far more theses have been written on the works of T. S. Eliot and E. M. Forster, who wrote very little and whose entire work can be read in a week, perhaps even less. Writers who are prolific are not greatly liked these days, but of course in the old days it was the nature of a writer to write much. Dickens, Thackeray, Balzac and Arnold Bennett all wrote many books. H. G. Wells always published at least four books a year, but this old image of the fecund, prolific, vital writer has disappeared in our own age. I think E. M. Forster did a great deal to kill the image.

Apart from writing rather a lot, I'm also a serious musician and a not very good painter; I discovered fairly early in life that I was colour blind, and I don't think this is good in a painter. I'm also a linguist, in that I'm interested in language. I think that language is probably the greatest human achievement. We use it every day, but we don't think about it. We use this mouth of ours and the air we breathe out, our teeth, our tongue and so forth, which are intended for quite different purposes, to create a series of symbols that can express the whole universe. This is the most remarkable thing in the world, raising us above animals. I marvel at this phenomenon daily, and I'm interested to see how it's manifested in different parts of the world, from China through to the Red Indians. Language is fascinating – I'm not a very good linguist myself in the conventional sense, but I find the linguistic pheno-menon remarkable.

For some time I was an education officer in Malaya and Borneo, and I have always enjoyed teaching. It is a very important job, and more satisfying than writing because you see a response to your work immediately. If you write a novel, especially in Britain, you throw it into a great silence, and there's no real response except the paid one of the critics and the newspapers. I don't know what effect a book is having on people except very, very occasion-ally. The Americans write to authors far more than the British do, because the British are very reserved about this kind of thing. I like to know what people think about my books, but I hardly ever hear. With teaching, however, you get this immediate response to your words, so you can check how they are going down and whether your meaning is being taken in. You can see people actually growing, becoming more adult and more mature, and take a tremendous pride in knowing that it is all through your own work, your own use of language, your own use of ideas, and so on.

I have been asked whether I use words intricately in order to express deeper meaning, or whether I write books in order to be able to use words intricately. I think that all writers have their different styles. Somerset Maugham had a very simple style of writing which made him a very popular writer – people like sim-plicity for the most part. However Maugham made the great error of supposing that this was the best way to write and the only way to write. It's a matter of temperament. I was brought up on music, so I'm tremendously interested in the patterns words can make. At the same time I recognize that human nature is too complex and contradictory for any simple language to express the human mind and temperament. The language you use to express this must therefore be complex and ambiguous.

My recent novel *Earthly Powers** has a homosexual for its central character. To some extent it was a kind of discipline to write as something totally different from myself, but I feel it's the job of the novelist to be able to enter the skin of all people. It should be possible for a male novelist to create credible women and vice versa, and of course women *have* created credible men from Jane Austen on. I was in America a short while ago, conducting a terrible institution they have there called a creative writing class – they believe that writing can be taught. Some of the black people in the class said that no white man could create a black character, some of the women said that no man could create a woman, and so on. I felt that this was totally false; we are human beings, all members of the same tribe and members of each other. It's a writer's job to try at least to penetrate into a mentality he doesn't fully understand or thinks he doesn't fully understand . . . to try and force himself to understand it.

I don't know what the homosexual temperament is really like except from the outside. I don't know what homosexual sensations are like. But one has to make the effort, to dare risking possible failure to present it. My choice of a homosexual was partly that, and partly also that I needed a character who was aware of a division in himself. He was a Catholic and also a homosexual, thinking to himself that God had made him homosexual and yet the Church, which is supposed to be the voice of God, was telling him that it was a sin to be homosexual. The consequent dilemma he finds himself in is of course very useful to me as a writer, because I can present conflict and his attempts to resolve it. Of course he can't resolve the conflict except by becoming an old man and ceasing to have any sexual instincts; then he can go back to the Church. This in itself is not much of a story, but it's the framework for a much bigger story, about free will, how far we are responsible for what we are or what we do, and what God is all about – this curious, enigmatic entity we call God, whose intentions we can never really devise. It's all about the unknown ability of God on one level – and of course on another level it's meant to be an entertainment, a diversion.

*Published by Hutchinson

GERRY FITT

The Independent MP for North Belfast and his wife explain what life is like for a politician and his family in that troubled province

One of the main arteries into Belfast from the north is the Antrim Road, and just before it spills its traffic into Carlyle Circus there's a depressingly run-down area where many of the terraced houses are bricked up. On one side are the remains of a hotel burned in the early 1970s and not rebuilt. On the other side is number 85, trim and well painted, but enclosed in wire netting and bullet-proof glass, with a television camera trained on the front door, which shows signs of attention from people who believe that the brick is mightier than the word. This is the home of Gerry Fitt, co-founder and leader of the SDLP until 1979, and now Independent MP for West Belfast. He talked about what it's like running a constituency surgery under such conditions.

'A lot of the people who come here are strangers to me – not even from my own constituency, but from all over Northern Ireland. So if I look through the spy hole in my front door and I see a man or a woman, I often don't know who they are. It's an awful thing to say, and I don't like the fact, though I have to live with it, but I have a revolver or an automatic pistol in my pocket; I open the door and have to make up my mind very quickly whether they're genuine or not. It's something that an English or Scottish or Welsh MP would find very hard to understand.'

Vast numbers of people file through what Gerry Fitt calls his confessional. Mostly they come from his sprawling West Belfast constituency, but when *Woman's Hour* went to see him the people in his waiting-room included four from other constituencies, and there was a surprising mix of Roman Catholics and Protestants. 'This is my daughter,' said one of them, 'and I've come to talk about a problem concerning her and our housing. I have her four youngsters, all living together.' She described Gerry Fitt as '. . . the only one who will do anything for any person, no matter what denomination they belong to.'

Gerry Fitt himself expanded on this. 'Very fortunately, through-out my political life I have represented people of all religions and of none, and once you get a name for having helped someone, they will tell their relatives or friends who are in trouble. But there is that great distinction, that in Northern Ireland you represent people who seek your assistance, and you don't pay attention to the geographical area in which they live.'

The problems brought to Northern Ireland's MPs are very similar to those experienced anywhere in the United Kingdom. Mostly they concern housing, or welfare benefits. A young couple who were squatting were seeking help after the owner of the house had arrived, threatening to shoot them. 'We got some threatening phone calls,' the man began, 'and then on Wednesday night he came in where me and my wife were and he produced a gun. So I got the police and all that, and they said it was a legally held fire-arm.' He still shouldn't have threatened them with it, though. It's not legal to do that!

Nearly every problem has a specific Northern Ireland twist to it, however. The bricklayer trying to claim sickness benefit was convalescent after being shot in his bed the previous autumn. The painters who sought advice about unfair dismissal lived in a Republican district and had refused their firm's instructions to carry out a contract at a police and army base, fearing that they would be intimidated and used to carry explosives. Then there was a butcher who was being forced to pay protection money to a paramilitary organization.

Gerry's own life has given him the sympathy to tackle anything. He went to sea at fifteen, and talked about his time in the Mer-chant Navy, in which he served throughout the Second World War, and the way it influenced his political ideas. 'That in fact was where I developed some of my political thinking. I remember my first convoy in 1942, going up to Murmansk in Russia on a tanker. The Royal Navy were dropping depth charges all round the convoy in an attempt to get the German submarines, because a wolf pack of U-boats was attacking it. I remember standing and consciously thinking, "Now what's this all about? Who are the fellas down there in submarines, trying to kill me? If they hit this ship they'll certainly succeed. There are a lot of Royal Navy men, too, and they're dropping depth charges, trying to kill the Germans in the submarines." I recall building up from that minute a dislike for nationalism as such. I would like to see Ireland united because I am a socialist. I don't like nationalism as a creed – I think it is a very destructive force. As the war went on, and particularly after the war ended, I saw an awful lot of poverty. I remember seeing terrible, grinding poverty in Jamaica – it had an awful effect on me, and I began to develop political philosophies and ideals, which is what got me into politics in Ireland.'

Irrespective of their ideology, Irish politicians are often the targets of violent dissent. Some have died; some have survived. Gerry Fitt, too, has had many attacks on his home and his person, the worst being in August 1976. 'At four o'clock in the morning', he said, 'they arrived, and began to throw a lot of stones and bricks. There were two or three hundred of them, and it was a very nasty situation. In the meantime I was speaking to police headquarters with a two-way transmitter which I have, and my wife was making telephone calls. The crowd grew steadily more intense and more vicious, until at twenty-eight minutes past four precisely – and that was an awfully long half-hour – they succeeded in pushing the door off its hinges. They raced right up the stairs into the bedroom where Ann and myself and my young daughter, who had come in from her own bedroom because she was very frightened, were. She opened the door and said, "Daddy, they're coming up the stairs!" It was a really bad mob. I grabbed a revolver from beside the bed, and stood and stopped them at the top of the stairs, on the very last step before coming into the bedroom. It was a period of two or three minutes when anything could have happened, an occasion that I am not likely ever to forget. Had I not had a revolver the crowd would certainly have been in and would probably have had Ann. They might not have realized what they were doing – many of them had been drinking or had taken drugs.'

Guns, bodyguards and security have become an integral part of the Northern Ireland politician's lifestyle, and it's an essentially lonely existence. Gerry Fitt spends more than half the week away from home on parliamentary duties; he needs to travel fast – although he admits to being afraid of aeroplanes, and says he's a better Catholic at 29,000 feet than he is on the ground; and his home is ever open to people in need of assistance. There's little privacy, and it takes a very special relationship for a politician's marriage to survive all that; Ann Fitt's stoicism and humour underpin the Fitt partnership. 'We're never apart in spirit for a start,' she said, 'and there is the telephone, which we avail ourselves of at every opportunity – Gerry usually rings me three or four times daily. I know he's going to be home at the weekend – and in any case there's always so much to be done here.'

'I think someone said to me,' said Gerry, 'very early in my political career, that the only one you should really depend on is your wife, because someone who may be your political friend that day could be your political enemy by the end of the week. Political friendships are not really lasting, which I have found throughout my political life. In 1972 there was a very nasty atmosphere prevailing in Northern Ireland. A lot of people were being murdered, and a lot of local authority representatives were withdrawing from Parliament because they were under intimidation from paramilitary forces. A vacancy came up in the local government area which I then represented; there was tremendous pressure from the party of which I was then a member, the SDLP, not to fight this seat, and there was also tremendous pressure from paramilitary gunmen who said that if we did decide to fight the seat they would kill the candidate and cause all sorts of disruption. Everyone that I had opposed was frightened to fight the election, and I didn't want a non-opposed return to be given to my political opponents. This was just more than flesh and blood could take, so far as I was concerned. I went to the City Hall, took out nomination papers and filled in a name. I then rang up my wife and told her that I had succeeded in getting a candidate to fight the election. Then I told her that it was a woman candidate, and she replied, "That's even better." I said, "Wait till I tell you her name." It was Ann's name that I had put on the nomination papers. So she was a candidate, whether she liked it or not. In fact she went into that election and won it hands down, but that was one time when Ann and I stood against everyone else.'

Ann dutifully held that seat for ten months until the circumstances had changed. But she prefers to take a back seat; she has asthma, and over the past decade has suffered severely each time a mob has hurled futile though very real abuse at the home she and Gerry have built up together. But she speaks for both of them when she says that the daily missiles are more than compensated for by the feeling that she and Gerry can genuinely help people in difficulty. 'Sometimes I sit down and I feel a bit of a martyr. I think, "Bless us and save us, is this never going to end? Is this the story of my life?" And I feel it would be great if we could go away some place and not have to worry about people's problems, or not have to listen, or not have to bother. But then I just settle down and get on with it.

CRYSTALLIZED FRUIT FROM TINNED FRUIT

Sally Tarrant-Willis, Crafts Editor of Reader's Digest, *gives a recipe that makes a delicious Christmas present. It involves a process lasting several days, but is well worth the effort*

1 large can pineapple, apricots or peaches
at least 12 oz (350 g) granulated sugar

Tip the fruit with its syrup into a bowl. If there is not enough syrup to cover the fruit, make more by melting sugar in water in the proportion of 8 oz (250 g) sugar to 7 fl oz (200 ml) water. Put a plate on top of the fruit to keep it submerged, and let it stand for 24 hours. Pour off the syrup into a pan, add 2 oz (60 g) sugar, bring to the boil and pour back over the fruit. Leave to stand for another 24 hours. Repeat twice. Put the fruit and its syrup in a pan, add 3 oz (90 g) sugar, and boil for 3 to 4 minutes. Place in a bowl and leave for 48 hours. Repeat until the syrup is like thick honey. Now leave to soak for 3 days. At the end of this time remove the pieces of fruit from the bowl, place on a wire rack, and dry in a very cool oven until they no longer feel sticky. Keep the fruit away from the sides of the oven or it will stick and burn. Pack the fruit pieces in layers, separated by waxed paper. Do not seal the package or make it airtight, or the fruit may go mouldy.

SPICED ORANGES

Excellent with cold meats and an ideal accompaniment to what's left of the turkey after Christmas. Another unusual Christmas present idea from Sally Tarrant-Willis, they need a month or so to mature

12 large oranges
1 pint (600 ml) white malt vinegar
2½ lb (1 kg) granulated sugar
1½ sticks cinnamon
¼ oz (7 g) cloves

Wash but do not peel the oranges, and slice them about ¼ inch (5 mm) thick. Put the slices in a pan and barely cover with cold water. Simmer, partly covered, until the peel is tender. Put the vinegar, sugar and spices in another pan and bring to the boil to make a syrup. Drain the oranges, keeping the liquid. Put half the oranges in the syrup. Cover and simmer until the oranges turn clear – about 30 to 40 minutes. Lift the oranges out. Put the rest in the pan and cook as before. If necessary, add some of the orange liquid to cover the slices if the syrup level falls. If the syrup is not thick at this stage, pour it off and boil until it thickens. Then add the orange slices and reboil. If the syrup is thick enough, merely heat it slowly, with the oranges, to boiling point. Pot in warm, sterilized jars. If there is not enough syrup to cover the orange slices in the jars, make some more, boil until thick, and fill up the jars. Keep for 5 to 8 weeks before eating.

SHOPLIFTING

Three people in very different situations talk about their experiences. First, a young girl who stole for fun explains in her own words why and how she did it, and what happened afterwards

We went into Marks and Spencer's. That's the most daringest place of the lot – it's got store detectives and that, 'cos we've heard about that at school. So we looked at the cashmere – the most expensive – and we thought, 'Ooh, that looks really nice.' I was feeling it for a little while, then we walked around with a couple of jumpers. You pick the stuff up and just pretend you're going to find an empty pay desk. Then you happen to put it in your bag or up your skirt or something, and you carry on walking. But someone tapped me on the shoulder – it was like one of them films, and you don't know whether to run or just stay there. One of my friends ran, and I was calling out to her, 'Sara, it's not worth it, 'cos they're going to run you down and I'm in trouble.' I was mostly thinking about myself – it's a bit weird, but you do think about yourself as well.

They searched my bag afterwards, and there was a whole pile of clothes and all sorts on the table. We didn't even realize how much we'd got. We were more shocked than what they were, I think. After that the Black Maria was outside, and this really shit us up a bit. They opened the door and banged it – they want to scare you. In a way it's a good thing, because you think, 'Gosh, I'm not going to do this thing again.'

My Mum was the first one to arrive. That's the worst thing you can imagine. You think, 'Gosh, my Mum seeing me in a cell.' She was in tears and that got me in tears, and everything was all soppy and really horrible. And that scared me for life, I think.

At the Juvenile Court you hear them say, 'You know why you're here. . . .' They always say that, I don't know why, and you have to say, 'Yes, sir.' And they say, 'Well, we're going to let you off *this* time', and so it makes you think that they're giving you this chance, so don't mess it up again. Everyone just seems to repeat themselves. 'Don't do it again, will you?' 'Well, we don't want any more trouble from you, do we, young lady?' (It's always 'young lady'.) The social worker, she's like saying, 'Well, why did you do it?' And I said, 'I dunno.' But she expected more. I said I didn't know, I'm a thick kid, and really you *don't* know. But she went on saying, 'Well, are you gonna do it again?'

Now how can I tell the future? They ask you these really stupid questions – it's just interference, what they're doing. If you've got sensible parents, when they've taught you, that's enough. My friend who was still doing it just got beaten and sent to bed. My Dad was telling me that it's not worth it, and saying you've got to think of your career, and he went on, 'What would you do if you got married, and you know that you've got to keep on nicking for your support, and this guy might be using you . . . ?' You know, my Dad was talking sense. I really appreciated that.

Yvonne Gunn tells a frightening story about how easy it is for the innocent to be convicted for shoplifting

My daughter didn't meet me at the station as we had agreed, and I thought she'd got held up in the traffic. Since she was obviously going to miss that train, I went home anyway and in due course met the next one. She was absolutely distraught. 'Don't smile', she said, 'I've been in a police station.'

I couldn't believe it, and said, 'What do you mean?'

'They say I stole something,' she replied, 'and I've been all this time in a police station.'

What had happened was that as she left a shop she heard a noise which she didn't take any notice of, walked along the pavement, and was stopped. A young man said, 'Will you come back? I think you have something in your bag which you haven't paid for.' He made her put the bag through the alarm system, and sure enough it sounded. Then he opened the bag and there was a jacket.

'I didn't put it there', she said.

And he said, 'That's rather a silly story. I'm sure you did.'

She had been in that shop for perhaps forty minutes, trying on a jacket in the changing-room, very similar to the one found in her bag. Foolishly she put her own carrier bag on the floor and then walked up and down looking at herself in the mirror from this angle and that. Then she tried another jacket on. . . .

Anyway, she was taken into the security office where they were rather nasty and said, 'You'd better make up a better story than that. You must have taken it. How did it get there?'

All she could think of was, 'I didn't do it. I didn't put it there.'

'Well, think of something better,' they kept saying to her, 'or we'll send for the police.'

She got the impression that if she had said, 'Yes, I did do it. I'm sorry, I'll pay', they would have let her off. But I believe that they wouldn't have done that. She stuck to her story, though, and just said that she didn't know about it.

So they sent for the police, and my daughter went off in a police van, which she said was very frightening. On the way they stopped at another shop to pick up somebody else. By now she was with two policemen, who questioned her all the time, and asked her why she had done it. She said, 'I didn't', and then they asked what her parents did, what her father did, telling her how horrible it would be when it got into the papers, and how bad it would be for her mother when other people read it. They leaned on her fairly heavily, and I think she felt very miserable, but she just said, 'I'm sorry. I didn't do it.'

My own first reaction when she told me the story was 'Now, did she do it?' So I asked her, and she said, 'No, I couldn't do that.'

I said, 'Are you sure it's not a joke? Perhaps somebody at school dared you to take something?'

'No, don't be silly,' she replied. 'I just couldn't do something like that. I would be too frightened.'

Then I believed her, because she's never lied and she's a sensible girl. I was naive in expecting to convince other people of her innocence, though. We had two options – trial by jury, or the magistrates' court – and we chose the latter.

It was at Great Marlborough Street, which I believe is very busy with cases like this. I thought our solicitor made quite a good case, saying that, though nothing could be proved, the girl had a good reputation so far and ought to be given the benefit of the doubt. But the magistrate just said, 'I find you guilty', and then, 'This is a sad case.' I'm sure he says that quite a lot, but it doesn't really help. The jacket was produced, and she tried it on in court. It was obviously too small and didn't fit her at all across the shoulders, but the magistrate didn't look.

The sentence was a £25 fine and £50 costs, and we went back feeling dirty and dreadful. I didn't care what other people thought, but I did care that she hadn't been believed. Then five days later the court rang up and asked us to come back. I asked why, and they said that the magistrate was reconsidering his sentence. So we went back.

The magistrate said to my daughter, 'I've thought about you a lot. I know you'll be looking for a job next year, or you might wish to travel, and this sentence will lie on your record. So I'm going to change it and give you a twelve months' conditional discharge. If you don't do it again in twelve months it will be wiped away.'

We felt glad in one sense, but in another sense worse, and I thought to myself, 'I think he's had doubts, and yet we're still left with a guilty verdict.' However at that moment we decided to accept things, because it was her A Level year. She was very shattered by the whole performance, and really didn't look herself. We were told we had three weeks in which to appeal, but she said she never wanted to go to court again. 'We can't ask you to,' I said, 'because you've got so much work to do this year.'

But the more we thought about it, the more angry we felt, and towards the end of the three weeks she said, 'I feel very angry about this case.'

'Enough to appeal?' I asked.

'I think so', she replied.

That appeal was postponed twice, which was heartrending, because each time she got very worked up, and the second time they only rang up the day before. Then she did her mock A Levels, which were disastrous – she's never done such bad exams before – and she was being sick, too. We didn't tie that up at the time, and just thought she had got a bug, but looking back now I'm sure it was caused by all the tension.

At last the appeal came to court. By then we'd got a barrister. In the meantime we had found a witness who said that sometimes children, for kicks, put things in people's bags, especially old ladies' bags. They watch the victim going out and have a good laugh when they see the terrible uproar and the person being upset and protesting. The other thing they sometimes do, apparently, is to put something in a bag which they want you to carry out for them; then they jostle you in the street and take it away, and you perhaps never know that you've carried it out for somebody else. This witness was believed, and we won the appeal.

I think my daughter is just about back to normal now. She's more cheerful, she's working hard, and she doesn't mind people asking her about it, although I think she would like eventually to forget all about it. When it was all over, she came and said thank you, which was wonderful because I had worried so much that we had put her in a difficult situation instead of forgetting about it. We had dragged it out for another six months. If we had lost that appeal I don't know what I would have done.

What makes otherwise respectable and honest people, particularly women, shoplift? The middle-aged listener who describes her traumatic experience below wrote a letter to Woman's Hour, *in which she said:* '[*It*] *included the first horror at realizing my action and of course the ordeal of prosecution, court appearance and sentence, and, perhaps more, the fear of a report in the local press. I had some knowledge, theoretically, of stealing as a symptom of emotional distress, but at sixty I was shocked to recognize that this could happen to me.*'

I was coming home from feeding a neighbour's cat. I'd promised to do this while she was on holiday, and on the way back I just casually thought I would stop and get some shopping. I should say that I was in a very depressed state, and had been for ten days or so. I went into the shop – an ordinary, self-service grocer's shop – and put a few things into a wire basket. I can remember thinking, 'Oh dear, all those cats to cope with', and I took four tins of cat food and put them straight into my own shopping basket. I knew what I was doing, and yet I think at that time if anyone had asked me if I was stealing I would have been shocked.

I went on, and I can remember seeing dried fruit and sultanas and thinking to myself, 'Oh dear, soon there will be all the apples to cope with, and I will have to make chutney. I can't cope.' I took a packet of sultanas, and similarly put those into my own shopping basket. I picked up something else – I think it was marmalade – but I put this in the wire basket, together with something else which I don't remember. I then took a packet of coffee, and don't remember if I had any specific thought about it as I had about the cat food and sultanas.

I went to the checkout, and I remember putting my own basket, in which the stolen things were, on the ground. I put the wire basket up and the assistant said to me, 'Would you like me to put them in your own basket?' And something within me said that this was my last chance, and that I'd been seen. But I just smiled and said, 'No, thank you. It's all right, I'll do it.' I paid for the things in the wire basket and put them into my own basket, and went outside. At that point of course a store detective, as I after-wards knew her to be, asked me to go back into the shop. I can remember very clearly being strongly aware of her black jacket and having a terrible sense of bitterness; somehow her jacket epitomized everything. I also had in my mind the thought of my mother's death many, many years before. Outwardly I was very calm, almost blasé, and I remember consciously thinking, 'I've got

to get through this. There has to be a way. You must play an act.'
I knew I had to pretend that I was someone else, and that I was
watching this person in order to put the character into a novel
which I would write.

Through all the proceedings and the police being called and
formal prosecution being made I was very calm, until I came out
from the police station with the official notice to attend court in
three weeks' time.* At this point I was aware of being physically
very shaky and feeling sick, but I knew I must get home. I drove
the car back and just went in and sat – I live alone. . . . I knew I
must do something, but I couldn't think of anything to do. Somehow the night went and in the morning, though physically I felt
very unwell, I think I was a little more reasonable about the whole
situation in the sense of recognizing that there was something very
wrong with me.

*When she appeared in court she pleaded guilty and was fined £100. The case
was not reported in the press, and she now sees a psychiatrist once a month

GINGERBREAD

Mary Berry's recipe makes a really sticky, dark, old-fashioned gingerbread

1 level teaspoon mixed spice
1 level teaspoon bicarbonate of soda
2 level teaspoons ground ginger
8 oz (250 g) plain flour
3 oz (90 g) lard
4 level tablespoons black treacle
4 level tablespoons golden syrup
2 oz (60 g) soft brown sugar
2 oz (60 g) chunky marmalade
2 eggs
6 tablespoons milk

Grease and line with greased greaseproof paper an 8 inch (20 cm)
square tin or a $7\frac{1}{2} \times 9\frac{1}{2}$ inch (19 × 24 cm) meat roasting tin. Pre-
heat the oven to 325°F (160°C, gas mark 3). Sift the spices,

bicarbonate of soda and flour into a large mixing bowl and make a well in the centre. Place the lard in a saucepan with the treacle, syrup and sugar and heat until the lard has just melted and the ingredients are blended. Draw the pan from the heat and cool slightly. Chop the marmalade roughly and beat the eggs. Stir the marmalade, eggs and milk into the bowl made in the flour. Then add the lard mixture, and beat with a wooden spoon until the mixture is smooth and glossy. Pour into the prepared tin and bake for 1 to 1¼ hours. Leave to cool in the tin for about 30 minutes, then turn out, remove the paper, and finish cooling on a wire rack. Eat on the day that it is made, or store in an airtight tin for at least a week.

THE ARRIVAL OF BENTLEY

Helene Hanff

Just before I left for London in October I got a note in the mail. 'Dear Miss Hanff,' it said. 'My sisters in England listen to your *Woman's Hour* broadcasts which make them feel they know what our life is like, since you live on East 72nd Street and my wife and I live on East 74th Street. The purpose of this note is to invite you to our block party on Saturday.'

I went to the block party, but this is the first chance I've had to deliver a message to his sisters from the gentleman who wrote the note. The message, from brother Henry on East 74th Street to his sisters Elizabeth in St Albans, Amelia in Clapham, Mary in Westminster, Victoria in Suffolk and Sarah in Sussex, is that the block party was a huge success. The block was closed to traffic for the day and the street and sidewalks were jammed with stalls selling T-shirts and sweaters and jewellery and china ornaments and plants and pillows and paintings and old books, in a giant white elephant sale.

But the main attraction of a block party is always the food. There were Japanese teriaki and sizzling Italian sausages and shish kebab and great plates of pâté and Brie. But most popular of all were the tables where residents of the block sold their own home-made specialities. Henry wants you to know he made a double batch of scones (pronounced as in 'bomb'); we Americans firmly call them scones (as in 'stone'). A mother and daughter made Alsatian *crêpes* with assorted fillings, and there were home-made cookies and brownies and carrot cakes and apple pies to take home for dinner.

The party ended with a raffle in which practically everybody won one of the prizes donated by local business people: a pair of movie tickets, dinner for two at the corner restaurant, a haircut and shampoo for the family dog, and so forth. Henry's American wife Patricia was treasurer, and told me that the block party raised nearly 7000 dollars to be spent on trees. Just trees? Well, first the committee will hire a contractor to uproot and cart away the block's diseased and dying old trees. Then they'll hire a nurseryman to sell them the ten new trees he thinks will grow best in small plots of earth on city sidewalks. When the trees are planted an expert bricklayer will be hired to build brick walls around them – high enough on the sidewalk side to keep out dogs, low enough on the gutter side to provide a run-off after rain. And finally a florist will advise which flowers will grow best in beds at the base of each tree. So now Henry's sisters have a full report on the block party.

Tomorrow is Thanksgiving and I'm pleased to report that my dinner guests will include an Old English sheepdog. Richard, owner of Chester, the sheepdog who died two years ago, drove out to the kennels last year to see about getting a new pup. He ordered his pup, but he saw a sight at the kennels which depressed him. A massive, full-grown Old English sheepdog was kept in a cage barely big enough for him. He'd been living in that cage for three months. The dog's name was Bentley, and for the first two years of his life he had lived with a family in Vermont. Then the family had to move to England for a year, and rather than quarantine Bentley there for six months they decided to leave him behind. They drove to the kennels, said to the breeder, 'Find a good home for him', and drove off. Bentley couldn't believe that his family had abandoned him. When he was locked in the cage he went berserk, tearing at the steel wire and barking until he was worn out. Finally he just gave up.

When Richard saw him Bentley was sitting in the cage hour after hour staring at nothing, as motionless as the wood. Richard pitied him, but he didn't want him. Nobody wanted him. Everybody wanted a pup. On a Saturday afternoon in September Richard drove up to the kennel to get his pup and when he got back he phoned me.

'Did you get your pup?' I asked. 'What's his name?'

There was a pause. 'Bentley', said Richard. 'I warn you, he's a nurd – he just sits. But I couldn't stand leaving him in that cage.' He added that Bentley had come alive enough to go over every inch of his new home with his nose, so there was hope.

'Bring him up', I said.

Richard came up a few minutes later accompanied by the most beautiful Old English sheepdog I had ever seen, with a thick, snow-white coat and enormous, snow-white paws. I sat in my

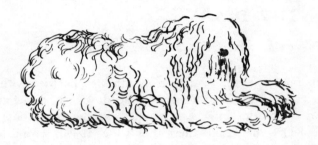

armchair and, at Richard's command, Bentley sat at my feet but with his profile to me. His face, entirely hidden under a mop of white fur, stared at nothing. I leaned down and, peering into the face I couldn't see, told Bentley he was the most beautiful sheepdog in the world. I told him there were lots of dogs in the neighbourhood who would be overjoyed to meet him. I told him he was going to be very happy in his new home with Richard and that all the people who lived in the building were going to admire and appreciate him. He sat unmoving, with no sign that he heard me. Finally I ran out of things to say, and stopped talking. I looked at Richard and sighed, and Richard shrugged. . . .

And Bentley offered me his paw.

WINTER

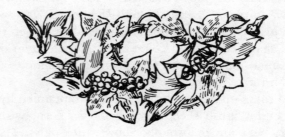

COUNTRY DIARY

Robin Page on the countryside in the Christmas season

December was another variable month weatherwise with wind, frost, rain and sun. We had some mild days, too, and bats were flying at dusk after insects. It seemed wrong to see bats in the middle of December, but there they were. It was wrong, too, on 21 December, which is St Thomas's Day, the shortest day of the year. The old rhyme says:

> St Thomas grey,
> St Thomas grey,
> The longest night
> And the shortest day.

But in fact it wasn't a grey day at all – it was a very sunny, clear day and very pleasant. It was very pleasant on Christmas Day, too – sunny, though quite cold:

> Sun through the apple trees on Christmas Day
> Means a fine crop is on the way.

We shall have to wait until next harvest time to see if we get good crops and good apples.

The village started getting ready for Christmas several days early. The carol singers came round and actually stopped to sing some carols. Over recent years we have had hit-and-run singing – singing a line, then rattling the tin. But this year they stopped.

In the village school the nativity play was really excellent –

much better than the 'Play for Today' on television. It was given star quality by Joseph who had no front teeth. The birth of Jesus was most unusual: Joseph and Mary appeared to be settling down for the night when suddenly they sprinted off the stage. Then they came back manhandling the baby and put it in the straw, which to me seemed a truly miraculous birth. It had never been done quite like that before. King Herod was also remarkable because I think he had modelled himself on Hitler and was stamping about the stage. That's a name you should remember in twenty years' time – Ben Foster, a quite outstanding performance.

The horticultural Christmas party, an event to which I had never been before, was interesting with such games as Guess the Seed, which I thought was quite original. There were also more orthodox things such as Pass the Parcel and Musical Chairs, all to the accompaniment of punch containing a lot of home-made wine.

On the farm the approach of Christmas was less entertaining because it involved plucking the poor old cockerels ready for Christmas dinner. There we were with an old bath, and down floating all around us as if we were in a snowstorm. It is not a pleasant job at all, and in fact I have now got plucker's elbow. It's made worse for me because I don't really agree with the way that we rear our cockerels. They put on weight too quickly, which means that they stagger about on weak legs and some even have heart attacks before we reach Christmas.

To me this is immoral, but the farmer is in a great dilemma because he wants the money but he can only get these cockerels – you can't really call them cockerels as they have been so highly bred by the scientists that they are just walking, flapping lumps of meat. It's surprising to me that the Ministry of Agriculture or some other body doesn't control the scientists so that we can rear things humanely. So often people condemn farmers, but they are caught – if they don't rear these cockerels other people will, and all the housewife wants is a cheap meal which is what she gets, but to me it spoils Christmas because I think it's cruel.

I think what we do on Boxing Day is a much better idea. My brother goes with his gun and dog to get a pheasant or a duck, and that's a much more humane way of getting your dinner. However, the cockerels tasted all right at Christmas dinner.

Whenever we have game or poultry we have a thing called light pudding, which has been in the family for some time. We eat it

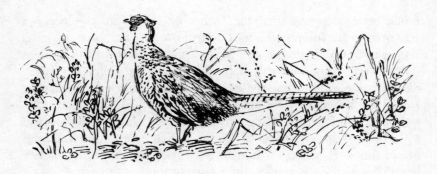

before the main course, with thickened gravy. You make it with eight ounces of self-raising flour, one teaspoonful of baking powder, three ounces of margarine, two eggs and some milk. The fat is rubbed into the flour, then the beaten eggs are added and mixed in. Finally the milk is poured in – the consistency should be quite stiff. The mixture is then baked in a greased dish for twenty minutes until it is risen and crisp. I don't know where this recipe comes from, but it starts the meal off extremely well.

And so Christmas passed. My poor nephew burst out crying after Christmas dinner because he had looked forward to Christmas for so long that he was worried because it was going too quickly and he wanted to start again. But I don't think many other people wanted to start again.

Yesterday I saw a fox. January is the month when foxes breed and so I expect to see them several times over the next few days and hear them at night. So really the last month has been a good one: except for the cockerels.

CHRISTMAS CAKE ICING

Mary Berry's recipe will ice an 8 inch round cake (see page 158)

ALMOND PASTE

4 oz (125 g) icing sugar
4 oz (125 g) ground almonds
4 oz (125 g) caster sugar
2 egg yolks

1 to 2 tablespoons apricot jam, melted
½ teaspoon almond essence
1 teaspoon lemon juice

Sift the icing sugar into a bowl, add the almonds and caster sugar
and mix well. Add the egg yolks and flavour with almond essence
and then lemon juice. Work the mixture into a small, smooth ball
by hand, but do not over-knead. Divide the almond paste into two
pieces, in proportion two-thirds to one-third. Cut out paper patterns of a circle to fit the top of the cake and a long strip to fit
round the sides. Lay these out on a flat surface and scatter them
with a little caster sugar. Roll out the smaller piece of almond
paste to fit the circle and the larger piece to fit the long strip
generously. For the sides, it helps to roll a long sausage shape of
almond paste, and then flatten it. Brush the top of the cake with

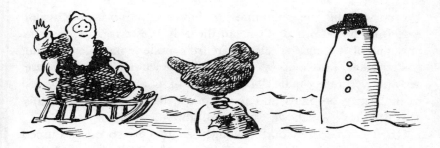

melted apricot jam, then put a circle of almond paste in position,
leaving the paper on. Turn the cake over. Brush the sides of the
cake with more jam, fix the strip of almond paste to the sides, and
remove the paper. Neaten the edges with a palette knife, and roll
a straight-sided tin around the cake to make the sides smooth.
Turn the cake back the right way up and put on a board. Remove
the paper from the top. Level the top with a rolling pin. Cover the
cake and leave in a cool place for 5 to 6 days to dry.

ROYAL ICING

1 lb (500 g) icing sugar
2 egg whites
2 teaspoons lemon juice
1 teaspoon glycerine

Sieve the icing sugar. Whisk the egg whites in a bowl until they become frothy. Add the icing sugar a spoonful at a time, then add the lemon juice and glycerine. Beat the icing until it is very stiff and white and will stand up in peaks. To ice the cake, thin down just under half the icing with a little egg white, mix to a spreading consistency and cover the top of the cake. Spread the remaining icing around the sides of the cake and rough up to form peaks. Keep a little icing, covered, in a cup, and use it next day to fix a candle and holly and ribbons on the cake.

KEEP OUT RUSSIAN FATHERS!

Bill Baker

I may well be the only male to have been inside a Russian maternity hospital. I don't mean the only Western male, but the only one of the male species apart from male gynaecologists and obstetricians, who 'belong' to this exclusive women's world. There are not even many male doctors – I think I saw one in four visits to maternity hospitals and to what the Russians call 'women's consultations', which we would call ante-natal clinics.

I had not realized that I would be breaking so many taboos when I asked to look at the subject of childbirth in the Soviet Union. The ordinary Russian male, even in his married state and even as a father, cannot get beyond the reception desk of a Russian maternity hospital. When I told the chief doctor of Moscow Maternity Home No. 64 that I had been with my wife while she was in hospital having our daughter she shook her head in horror. 'We don't allow that', she said. 'Men could bring in infection.' When I said that not only had I been in the maternity unit, but also I had been in the delivery room and assisted in the birth of my daughter, all present looked at me in utter disbelief. In fact, they decided that my Russian must have been at fault and that really I must have meant something else. No! I insisted, it really was quite the thing in England now for the father to be with the wife at the birth of their child and, despite differences between individual hospitals, it was usually possible. 'But what about the infection?' they asked. And I had a quick comic vision of this battalion of women doctors defending their charges against the infection of men!

No way can a Russian father get in to see his wife or baby. They can talk on the telephone, write each other letters, or, most usual of all, he can come round to the maternity home and, after inquiring at the official desk after the health of his wife and new baby, he can stand below the window of her ward, having alerted his wife by telephone beforehand. So it is that most Soviet men get the first glimpse of their newly born baby through a double-glazed window, usually two or three floors above their heads.

Inside, the medical attention which the Russian woman receives and the provisions made for her compare very favourably with the British National Health Service system. Indeed, in these days of health service cuts, in some things the Russians put us to shame. For instance, all women stay in hospital for five days after the birth to make sure they are rested and well before being sent home. The Russian maternity hospitals I visited were clean, well-equipped and efficient. The staff and doctors with whom I talked all seemed kind, caring people.

The social provisions are impressive. Since most women work in Russia, the four months' fully paid pregnancy leave is vital. If a mother wishes, she has the option of taking a full year off work to look after her new baby; the job will be kept open for her without loss of pay or status.

But husbands are not wanted. In some cases this can be particularly hard. By coincidence, friends of mine in Moscow have just had their first baby. Unfortunately Natasha, the wife, developed high blood pressure. With praiseworthy efficiency she was whisked into the maternity home straight away, a good two months before the baby was due. For two months Natasha was isolated from the outside world and her husband. And her husband was isolated from her.

What do Russian men think of this state of affairs? Are they in revolt against this hijacking of their wives by the Russian medical profession? Not at all. Just as, say, twenty years ago in Britain it was accepted that the place of the husband was in the corridor outside, pacing anxiously up and down awaiting the news, so Russian men seem to accept that giving birth is women's work. 'I wouldn't want to see my wife going through all that', was a typical comment. It exactly mirrored the comment of one of the women doctors I talked to, that 'It wouldn't be nice for a man to see his wife in labour. It could affect their relationship.' Of course my argument was: 'Quite right, it could affect their relationship – but only for the better!' But I did not get far with that one.

I wonder why it is that the important emotional aspect of childbirth is ignored? At the Moscow maternity hospital I mentioned that in many British maternity units the mother was encouraged to put the baby straight to the breast after delivery, before even the cord is cut. The Soviet doctor replied that they had heard of that and tried it, but had stopped since they found that there was little trouble in getting babies to take the breast anyway. I thought the reply was enlightening because she had seen only half the point. The more important part is that after the rigours of birth the mother, baby and husband should have time to 'be' before the impersonal medical routine takes over. The psychological aspect had just got lost.

I don't think that it is the Soviet medical profession which is at fault here. Sheila Kitzinger, in her book *Women as Mothers*,* remarks that '. . . in any society the way a woman gives birth and the kind of care given to her and the baby point as sharply as an arrowhead to the key values in the culture'. Communist culture stresses the full equality of women, but traditional Russian culture seems to me to have carried through to the present day the emphasis on the separate man's and woman's world. It's something that exists on a much deeper level than laws or slogans, and I think it's that which, as yet, makes it unthinkable for a Russian man to be with his wife in hospital at the birth of their child.

*Sheila Kitzinger talks about her views on childbirth on page 68. *Women as Mothers* is published by Fontana

BROOMBALL

Virginia Waite is a journalist and married to John Osman, the BBC's Moscow correspondent

Take one tennis court, add water and freeze. Repeat until the ice is thick enough to stand a dozen people, and what you have is a broomball pitch. The game evolved some twenty years ago in

Moscow, when a couple of bored British diplomats thwacked a child's plastic ball across the frozen embassy court with the nearest thing they had to hockey sticks – birch twig brooms used by the old ladies, the babushkas, who sweep the streets and gardens.

A kind of ice hockey was the result, but there are two significant differences from the real thing. Brooms, bound up with string and curved into a hook at one end, are used instead of proper sticks, and in place of skates the players, six a side, wear tennis or gym shoes which is what gives broomball its unique flavour. Rubber-soled footwear has to be the worst possible thing for keeping your feet on ice, and the game looks uncommonly like knockabout farce to the spectators.

The players consist of three forwards, two defenders and a goalie. Goals are of course scored rather more by accident than design, if a player happens to have slid in the right direction connected with the ball. The rules have been gradually amended to suit the skills, or otherwise, of the players. You can't touch the ball with your hands or kick it. The broom cannot be lifted above shoulder height, and it's definitely forbidden to bash your opponent in the face with it. Three referees are needed to oversee fair play. Persistent un-sportsmanlike behaviour gets you thrown off the pitch for two minutes.

The pastime has gathered all kinds of traditions and customs as well as teams, leagues and a fixture list of international games. It began as a men-only sport, but its growing popularity attracted women, too, who started playing some three years ago. The players range in age from eighteen to those in their forties, and are mostly embassy personnel and diplomats' wives whose children cheer them on from the sidelines. Despite the fact that some players bear the visible scars of broomball, its dangers tend to be minimized by its devotees.

Linda Campbell, a twenty-seven-year-old secretary, is the captain of the British women's team and she reckons the ladies measure their length rather less often than the men – or, put another way, more men break their bones than women, because they play more aggressively. Everybody wears the kind of protective clothing associated with American football players. There are elbow pads, and knee pads – very handy for using as sledges to launch a rugby-style tackle – and helmets to stop you from slitting your head open. Nothing, however, can prevent the bruised limbs that are the mark of the true broomball player, and as long as the ice holds, keen men and women can be seen falling about in Moscow every Saturday.

FASHIONS FROM MOSCOW

Virginia Waite

There isn't a button to be seen on the newest Soviet fashions – because buttons are scarcely to be found here. So Russia's leading designer sensibly omits them from his styles. Zippers are used sparingly and discreetly, too, for supplies are erratic and choice limited. In fact designer Slava Zaitsev uses only the simple materials that are actually on sale to everybody in the shops.

But long before he and the other sixty designers at Moscow's House of Fashion start even to think of next year's look they get together with the Aesthetic Committee of the Ministry of Light Industry. The Ministry lays down the production targets under the current plan. These include precise details of colours and prints for fabrics, trimming and accessories. The designers make their choice and only then begin to design the clothes.

When it comes to the finished product, marketing takes a very different turn from the West. Haute couture doesn't exist, and it would be politically unacceptable for people to have expensive custom-built clothes. Exclusivity is actually the last requirement.

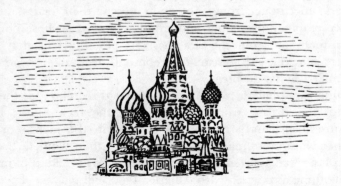

The major priority is clothes that are suitable for all, and at the right price. So the first to view the new collections are the clothing factory directors. They are free to modify or adapt the designs according to local needs and supplies. Those who can't reach Slava's showings work from the design book, published annually with illustrations. The latest line goes into mass production as the materials come off the looms and presses.

But Russians are very keen home dressmakers, too. And after the trade has seen what's new, Slava Zaitsev gives a public show to an invited audience. I saw at least a third of them busily sketching the clothes to make for themselves. First, however, they had to listen to a startling tirade from the designer about their lack of dress sense. He harangued them on what he called their 'unfashionable' fur hats for winter, and about the drabness of their wardrobe for the rest of the year. They often dress worse than peasants, complained Slava, but he made sure that everyone recognized the thin, silky black fur beloved by the peasants when it appeared in his show as an evening coat.

He reintroduced the mini in a handful of fun tunics, and had the models go barefoot, explaining that he hadn't yet got round to designing shoes, and that until he did so there was no suitable footwear to go with minis. The collection was equally divided between men's and women's clothes. Men's jackets had a casual blouson look to disguise the absence of buttons. The key to the women's outfits was high, squared shoulders. Most dresses had pleats or slits at the back and eye-catching bows and belts. Zippers were unobtrusively positioned or hidden, so that if they didn't match perfectly it wouldn't show.

The collection was – despite the emphasis on practicality – stunning and modern, echoing what the West showed a year or so ago. Zaitsev included lots of matching coats, because temperatures can be coolish here even in summer and almost everyone has to use public transport. He also had lots of matching pillbox or toque hats, to get away from the woolly headpiece that is the general alternative to the winter fur hat. Dress-and-coat outfits were classically elegant, with lavish use of material in wide skirts. They were displayed in two versions to show off to best advantage the limited colour combinations.

There are national costumes for each of the fifteen Republics in the Soviet Union, and Slava likes to present his contemporary version of these. The exotic south was obvious, in shocking pink evening pantaloons. It was the kind of theatrical touch for which Slava is known – when he joined the House of Fashion after a not-too-successful stint designing overalls and protective clothing in a factory, his more conservative colleagues protested that his work was too flamboyant. There's a grain of truth in this. The forty-year-old designer loves making clothes for the theatre, and was responsible for dressing the thousands of Soviet athletes and others who took part in the opening ceremonies of the 1980 Olympic Games. His latest attentive audience may not have been planning to break world sporting records, but the sewing machines will undoubtedly be whirring in the race to see who will be first on the scene with this season's fashions.

NATALIE WOOD

The American film actress talks about her life and career

I started off as a child actress and my first part was a very little one when I was four. A year later the man who had directed that picture had a rather larger role for a five-year-old, and remembered me. It was a film with Orson Welles and Claudette Colbert called *Tomorrow is Forever*, and I had quite a big part: they bleached my hair, and I had to speak German, as well as learn to speak English with a German accent.

My older sister was a movie fan and had scrapbooks in which she put the pictures she had collected, and I was quite a fan of Sonia Henje and John Payne, as I recall. So when I was told that I was going to go to Hollywood to make a screen test, in my imagination I thought it would all be golden and velvet and wonderful. The first disillusionment, of course, was seeing the rather ordinary-looking, barn-like sound stage where films are made. I remember that vividly and when, a few years later, I made a film called *Inside Daisy Clover*, I related to that feeling, which is how she felt at the vastness and bareness and 'oldness' of movie stages.

My background is Russian, and my real name is Natasha Gurdin. It was the producer of *Tomorrow is Forever* who gave me my present name. He thought that Natalie would be better and more easy to pronounce than Natasha; a friend of his was a director named Sam Wood, which I think is why he arbitrarily chose Wood. I was very upset because I thought Wood sounded awful, and I wanted it at least to be Woods, which conjured up a nicer mental picture to me.

Both my parents were born in Russia, but left when they were four or five years old. My father's family went to Canada and my mother's family to China, where she lived until she was about fifteen. They are both American citizens now, and I was born in San Francisco. But the Russian side of me was remembered a year or two ago when I was asked to do a television show in Leningrad about the Hermitage museum, which was shown on BBC Television. That was my first trip to Russia. It was most interesting because I had just done a film with Sean Connery in which I had to speak Russian and play a Russian interpreter. I did speak the language as a child, but in this film I had to speak with rather more sophistication than a ten-year-old, which was my age when we stopped speaking it at home. So I brushed up my Russian with some three months of lessons. By the time that the film was finished and I went to Leningrad, I felt that I was quite fluent.

I'm not sure how many people on the street in Leningrad knew who Peter Ustinov and I were, though I think they looked at us all because we were dressed so differently from them. I was wearing a fur coat, because it was cold at the time, and my husband was wearing blue jeans which they loved, and offered to buy off him! Had we realized, we would have brought more blue jeans to give away. They wanted records of singers, too, so we would go into the dollar stores where only the tourists are allowed, and buy Barbra Streisand albums as gifts for waiters and other people.

I had very mixed feelings about going back to this land of my ancestors. It was very sad in many ways because I was full of the Russia of Chekhov, Dostoevsky and Turgenev, and Russian gipsy songs and the stories that my parents had told me, and of course it's quite a different Russia now. One of the things that I found disappointing was that, although the buildings are beautiful, the churches are gorgeous, and of course the Hermitage and its works of art are just dazzling, the people dress in a plain, ordinary way that doesn't look indigenous to any country, and because of this they seem to have lost part of their heritage.

I've been in films for a very long time now, having started so young, and naturally one remembers some parts more vividly than others – not just playing them, but also getting them in the first place. *Rebel Without a Cause* was one example. I had been working for many years but in those days, although I was exactly the right age – fifteen, and the girl in that movie was supposed to be fifteen – it was considered the thing to cast somebody a little bit older than the actual character. There's a practical reason for this, too, which is that if somebody is over eighteen they don't need to have welfare workers and they are allowed to work longer hours. If you're younger than that you can only work four hours out of the eight, and three hours are allotted to school time. I loved the part and wanted to play it, but I had to make three or four screen tests before they were convinced that I looked old enough to be a teenager. In a sense I suppose I had been typecast with braids and they could only see me as a little girl.

I had battles of a different nature when I was put under contract to Warner Brothers, who wanted me to do lots of pictures that I knew did not have good scripts. So I went on strike for eighteen months. The studio wouldn't allow me to work anywhere unless I did these pictures, and it was a sort of impasse because I didn't want to do the ones that they wanted me to do. The person who really saved me was Elia Kazan, the director of *Splendour in the Grass*, because he insisted on having me in that picture. Even though Jack Warner was telling me that I'd never work again unless I did this other picture for him, he had to respect Kazan's wishes, and so my contract was settled at that point. All I wanted was the right to do one picture of my choice a year, and the first such picture that I was able to do was *West Side Story*, so it was lucky.

In my personal life I've married the same husband – Robert Wagner – twice, and though I don't know if I'd recommend it for everyone it's certainly been very nice for me. I think one of the things that makes it terrific for us is that very often two people meet at the ages that we met the second time, and only know from hearsay details of the other person's background, family, earlier life and so on. In my case, though, at the time that we were married the first time I knew his whole family and background, and he knew mine. During the time that we were apart we both kept in contact with one another's family, so there remained a kind of connection that was never broken.

I have two daughters, the younger of whom is just past the age I was when I first started acting. From time to time both Natasha and Courtney ask if there's a role of a daughter in something that

I'm doing; then they put in their bid and say they'll do it. A recent film I did had a part for a five-year-old child; Natasha tried to convince me that she could look five, while Courtney tried to convince me that she indeed was five. I explained to them that this role consisted of a lot of crying, even when they didn't feel like it, and being cold, and it didn't really mean getting out of school, just going to school without any friends. After I had painted this very unattractive picture they decided that they might as well just stick it out at school.

I've had various awards and nominations from the profession, but one that gave me a lot of fun was when Harvard University named me worst actress of the year. *Harvard Lampoon* gave me this accolade for my performance in *Inside Daisy Clover*, which I think as a matter of fact was particularly liked in Britain. In any case I decided that it would be fun to go; I asked if anyone had ever gone to accept this award, and no one ever had.

While we were in New York waiting to take the plane we got a telephone call from people who said they were from the *Harvard Lampoon*, saying that Senator Kennedy was arriving, or something, and would we mind taking an earlier flight – there are shuttle flights every half-hour. So we said we would, and took the earlier flight. What we didn't know was that it was the rival newspaper, the *Crimsons*. They had pretended to be the *Lampoon* and they actually kidnapped me from the other plane. Then they gave me a 'good sport' award. The *Harvard Lampoon* people didn't know where I was, and searched and searched. Eventually they found me and I was given the awful award which was a man painted gold, like an Oscar. I decided to accept it, as people sometimes do, with a speech to the effect that I was terribly touched by this honour, but of course an honour like this didn't belong just to me alone, and that I wanted to share it with all the people that it rightfully belonged to, like the writer and the director and all the other actors. . . .

GINGERBREAD MEN

Sally Tarrant-Willis's gingerbread men are popular with children. If you make a hole in each gingerbread man before baking, you can thread a ribbon through and hang them on the Christmas tree. The mixture can also be used to make the shapes for a gingerbread house

4 oz (125 g) brown sugar
4 oz (125 g) golden syrup
2 oz (60 g) margarine
1 tablespoon milk
8 oz (250 g) plain flour
½ teaspoon bicarbonate of soda
¼ teaspoon ground cinnamon
¼ teaspoon ground ginger

Pre-heat the oven to 325°F (170°C, gas mark 3). Melt the sugar, syrup and margarine in the milk in a pan, but do not let boil. Remove the pan from the heat and cool. Sift the flour, bicarbonate of soda and spices into a large bowl. Pour in the syrup mixture and stir well. Cool a little, then roll out about ¼ inch (5 mm) thick. Cut

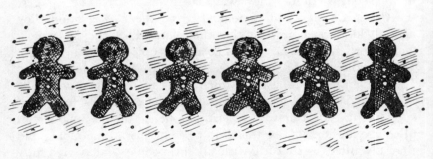

out the shapes with a special gingerbread man cutter, or, if you don't have one, use cardboard shapes which you can make yourself, and cut round them with a knife. Place on greased baking trays and bake for 15 minutes. Cool for 1 minute on the trays, and trim the shapes if necessary while they are still soft. Transfer to a wire rack to finish cooling. Decorate, if you like, with royal icing made from 1 egg white, ½ teaspoon lemon juice and 8 oz (250 g) sifted icing sugar (see page 205).

LOOKING AFTER WOODEN FURNITURE

Muriel Clark

What you do with your furniture depends on what kind of finish it has. Solid wood is the most expensive and the hardest-wearing, and you can do almost anything to it, because if it gets scratched or damaged you can sand off the top surface and repolish it. But most of the wooden furniture that we have now is chipboard with a veneer on it. You can always tell solid wood because the end grain – the grain at the edge of a piece of wood – will match the grain on the top, whereas in chipboard furniture the edge is usually a thin strip of wood glued on. You can tell by looking, but it's always wise to ask as well.

There's nothing wrong with chipboard furniture, however, if it's good quality. The best kind, with three layers, is much less likely to warp than cheaper kinds, and it does keep its shape very much better. Like everything else, you get what you pay for, but do ask in the shop. You won't always get advice, but the more people keep asking, hopefully the more likely they are to get information when they want it.

There are various finishes on wooden furniture. Furniture with a plastic surface only needs a wipe-over with a damp cloth. Teak furniture needs a rub from time to time with teak oil. In a centrally heated home teak does dry out very quickly, and this special oil will feed it. Don't, whatever you do, spray it with a silicone polish, because you'll spoil the lovely, dull, matt finish. Never use these polishes on matt-finished furniture, though they're fine for French-polished furniture or any shiny or painted surface. They're also very good for kitchen equipment – a fridge benefits from a spray with a silicone polish. If you've got real wax-polished furniture, which was wax-polished when bought, you should use a solid or liquid cabinetmaker's wax, which will give you that lovely old-fashioned patina.

While on the subject of surface finishes, there are a number of non-wooden ones about that are worth mentioning here. Painted furniture should be treated like any other paintwork – simply wash it over. It's a good idea to use a spray polish because it will bring back a nice shiny surface and it does help it stay clean. Plastic-finished furniture sometimes has grey marks when you buy it, and the insides of drawers develop these marks. The best thing to take them off is ordinary soap and water – make a lather and wipe it over with that. It lifts the stains off much better than any of the patent cleaners.

Accidental damage can hanpen in any home. Scratches, if not too deep, can be filled in with brown shoe polish. Iodine is useful, too, and some people recommend rubbing them with a walnut, which will restore the colour. You can buy special scratch cover polish which is very effective, and will also restore the colour to faded matt-surface furniture.

Furniture can be dented, particularly in a home with small children. The way to deal with minor dents is to steam them out with a damp cloth and a hot iron: the wood soaks up the moisture and the surface will rise again. However there isn't much you can do about a really bad dent.

Stains and marks are another frequent problem, and probably the commonest ones are caused by heat and burns. A surprising method of getting rid of heat marks is brass polish. It's very effective, though you do have to polish up the furniture again afterwards. For cigarette burns try a very fine steel wool and a little linseed oil, but if you really burn into the surface there's not a lot you can do. Wine and spirit marks are tricky to remove. Deal with them at once if you can – cooled cigarette ash rubbed into them sometimes does the trick.

One last piece of advice on this particular subject: if you have any kind of damage on a valuable antique, do get specialist advice before trying to tackle it yourself.

To remove a sticky build-up of polish on wax-polished furniture, wash it over with a cloth soaked in vinegar and water and then wrung out. If you have furniture with a lot of carving and curlicues, such as you find on some antique pieces, don't labour with a duster but use a nice soft brush or the brush attachment of your vacuum cleaner.

Always ask about furniture care when you buy – quite a lot of responsible manufacturers are now labelling their furniture. Do read the instructions, and then follow them; it's very important.

DO-GOODERS

Margaret Hollis

The term 'do-gooder' is usually used in a rather disparaging way. I don't really know why, because most of us know people who need our help. People who talk about do-gooding, too, often make it sound as if the person concerned just scattered benefits like confetti. In my experience it isn't like that at all.

I think the first thing we have to learn if we really want to help is to listen, not just to what people say, but to all the under-currents of feeling. We have to understand how a person can say one thing and mean quite the opposite, because somehow we've got to find out what they feel they need, not what we think they ought to have. Have you noticed how the best relationships seem to grow? We sometimes have the pleasure of taking on some small, daily job which a person can't do for themselves, and then finding ourselves accepted as friends. This is surely how do-gooding – such a horrible word – should end up, with both people benefiting, rather than patronage on one side and a burden of gratitude on the other.

One of the greatest difficulties, it seems to me, is encountered when we don't feel drawn to the person we're trying to help. As a friend said to me, 'I wouldn't mind kissing Auntie if only she didn't smell so.' Repulsion can be caused by people's characters, too, when we feel that part of their trouble stems from their selfishness or greed or unlovingness. It is difficult to feel in tune with them, and they probably find it a real effort to feel anything for us. Do-gooding may then become merely a matter of duty, and people can usually spot that a mile off. I once worked with a Church Army sister, and was impressed time and time again by her ability to find love and humour in the most unpromising situations and individuals.

How far does do-gooding take you, particularly in these days when social services are being reduced and doctors are over-stretched, so that there's more need for voluntary help? I once alerted a doctor to the possible need of one of his patients for treatment in a mental hospital. It took a lot of heart-searching, because I interfered. She was incapable of getting help for herself; she couldn't even change her clothes or wash, and her husband was knocking her about. Her doctor decided that hospital was indeed the answer. She had been there before and had made a good recovery. Unfortunately she didn't improve much, and although the doctors decided there was no point in keeping her in hospital, her husband, whom she still idolized, ill-treatment or not, wouldn't have her back. She is longing to go home, but it looks as if she's there for good. Perhaps if I hadn't intervened she wouldn't be there – or has her hospitalization saved her and her husband from real catastrophe? Would his violence have got worse? Where does proper concern stop and the old image of the officious neighbour begin? Perhaps it's right to say that we're on thin ice when we step outside our role of comforter and try to achieve things for our friends. On the other hand, what do you do when you think someone is at risk, as I did with her? I really don't know the answer to that one.

Do-gooding, it seems to me, is a question of a fine balance between doing too much and not enough, and of our knowing when we're in danger of tipping the scales. We need imagination – not too much, but enough to put ourselves into other people's shoes. I think it's true to say that the best comforters are usually those who have suffered themselves. Perhaps some of the people who make fun of do-gooders are seeking an excuse for themselves to stay clear of such commitments. I can say one thing. My experiences have made me more acutely aware than ever before of my shortcomings. Do-gooding isn't an easy option, whatever some people think. If we turned it round and just called it doing good, would it get a different image, I wonder?

LIFE WITH GOD

Sister Helen Simon talks about her life as an Anglican nun

What struck me most, at first, was that we had to be holy twenty-four hours of the day. I entered the order at a time when nuns were still being taught very traditionally, and the idea was that we should be in training, as it were, all the time, even when we were asleep. But I suppose what would strike an outsider most was the number of times we attended chapel every day. We keep a version of monastic hours, which means being in chapel for a service six or seven times a day. The First Office, as they are called, would start at 6.30. Before that we would have had an hour's silent prayer on our own. After the First Office we had Communion, and then breakfast. So we had been up for something like two hours before we had our first meal. I found it incredibly difficult to get used to because I'm very much a night person. One of the biggest shocks was getting up at 5.30 in the morning, and I felt exhausted by about nine at night. It was like a regression to childhood, having to go to bed so early. The other two main activities, very much on the Benedictine pattern, are manual work and spiritual reading.

For the first few years I did housework or worked in St John's Home, an old people's home that we run. I became very good at cleaning loos and baths, and one of the hardest lessons to learn was that whatever work you did wasn't important – it was the way you did it. My biggest fight was with boredom and monotony in the beginning. Gradually, as I got more established in the life itself, I began to be given tasks at which I was more naturally good – they tended to be more intellectual, I suppose. But now that I've taken my first vows and I've been transferred to the London house they've made me House Sister, of all the crazy things, which means I'm in charge of things like changing fuses and doing something with the boiler when it bursts. I had to teach myself what to do, so I went round to the local library and got out a book on electricity which I've been slowly plodding through. I think one of the most important things about a religious community, rather than a mixed community, is that the women have to fulfil the male function as well. You have to grow into your male side not only emotionally but also practically, because you have to do all the jobs that a mixed household would do.

My biggest problem when I first went into the convent was loneliness, because great emphasis is placed on solitude and silence. I also found it very hard to adapt to being a child again, in a way, because when you're a novice, as you're called, you have to go through all the emotional patterns of childhood and adolescence once more. It's a tremendously vulnerable position to be put into, and one with which you're really not equipped to deal. I am grateful now to have had the chance to go back and straighten out all the bent bits, but at the time I didn't quite see it that way.

There are of course many different orders and societies, and particularly since Vatican II there has been enormous outgrowth in communities. The Roman Catholics have gone into renewal in a big way, and the Anglicans are hopping along behind. But what happens in religious communities parallels what's happening in the Church as a whole. There's an emphasis on real sharing, on spontaneity, on cutting across all the social and racial barriers. But the main variation within religious communities centres on whether they are concerned with social work or whether they concentrate more on prayer and the enclosed style of life. I think our community is somewhere in the middle. We have a lot in common with other communities in the Church which do not comprise monks and nuns – for example, those interested in ecology. There are many different ways of being involved in the needs of the twentieth century and bringing a Christian slant to life, and we with our vows of poverty, chastity and obedience – the poverty one is uppermost – explore what it means not to waste food, how to use it constructively, and how to tie in with the needs of the Third World. I think religious communities have rather lost this awareness. They had it many centuries ago, but now it has passed to other types of community, and we need to get together and share our mutual insights so that we are really saying something to twentieth-century society, and aren't just some kind of lunatic fringe.

A number of generations are of course represented in our community, which, like many others in the Anglican Church, started in the Oxford Movement of the nineteenth century. There's a certain amount of consensus among the younger elements that we want to be much more of a voice in twentieth-century society, but as regards our position in the Church there are an incredible number of members of the Church of England who have never even heard of religious communities. So we have quite an enviable freedom to experiment within the structure of the Church. If we really grasp the opportunity we could be quite radical – almost pioneers. We could explore new lifestyles within Christian communities, for instance. We could explore liturgy, and in fact we are beginning to. In the last two or three years the community has changed unbelievably. A new Mother was elected just over two years ago, and her arrival coincided with an upsurge of revolutionary feeling, since when we've re-written our Rule of Life. We suspended the rules of silence while we explored what we really meant by silence, and individual sisters within the community

222

have been encouraged to resume their intellectual interests and to explore what it means not just to follow blindly a Rule of Life. A couple of sisters and I have become very involved in Jung; it's very interesting to me because I'm concerned with the whole question of the stereotype image of the nun, and the kind of looks you get when you're in the street. Sometimes you see contempt and sometimes you observe some kind of yearning in people's expressions, and I discovered from Jung that nuns carry a certain projection of purity and remoteness and a certain kind of ideal womanhood.

That's not exactly the way I feel, though I know what they are getting at. It's the attraction of the Holy Grail kind of symbolism, which was in fact part of the life's attraction to me, but when I entered the community I realized that you didn't leave the whole of your body or the rest of your personality outside. It's brought me up against different parts of my personality, which I probably wouldn't have come up against any other way. During the last four years I've really begun to grow into my own womanhood, for the very reason that I saw what it meant to have certain aspects denied – like, for example, the physical, sexual side. When that's removed you have to search for your essential womanhood and explore it spiritually, emotionally and intellectually. One of the things that's been most important to me is to discover that love in all its different forms – for men, friends, children and God – ultimately comes back to the same source, and I've even felt the same physical sensation in the pit of my stomach for different kinds of love. I've learnt that the feelings that I experienced previously, say during a love affair with a man, find an authentic expression in the prayer relationship with God. It can be so much like a love affair. The feelings are the same, but you discover their roots, buried far back in the whole reason why you were made, which I believe increasingly was primarily for a love relationship with God. All the other love relationships in one's life are aspects of that, and as I get older I see more and more the bigger picture which has God's arms around it.

A NEW YORK CHRISTMAS

Helene Hanff

Here are some potential gifts for the proverbial friend who has everything. The following items were taken from three American Christmas catalogues that had to be read to be believed.

Item No. 1 is from the Gucci catalogue. It's a lizard handbag and it has an eighteen-carat gold handle, which can be detached and worn as a necklace. So Gucci probably thinks it's a bargain at only $11,500.

Item No. 2 comes from the catalogue of Hammacher-Schlemmer, a home furnishing store like no other. For example, in these energy-shortage times the Hammacher-Schlemmer catalogue advertised not only an electric foot warmer and an electric fish scaler, but an electric record cleaner for your dusty record albums. Their prize gift in this catalogue is for the executive in your life. It's an electronic desk fitted out with an electric cigarette lighter, an electric pencil sharpener, an electric paper shredder, a digital clock, a digital thermometer, an electronic calculator, a radio, a cassette player and recorder, and a small colour TV set. All this for only $8,950, making it cheaper than the Gucci handbag. But of course, that's not including what the desk's ten electric gadgets will do to your electricity bill, which would turn even Gucci pale.

And finally, an item from Neiman Marcus, a famous Texas emporium which has opened a multi-million dollar store in a New York suburb. Their prize catalogue item is described as 'the Earth as only the astronauts have seen it'. It's a globe, revolving on a special base, and the globe and base together weigh 495 lb. If you can get it through your front door, and are willing to knock out a couple of walls to make space for it in your living-room, you can have it, personally delivered and installed by an expert, for only $14,500.

Never mind. All this insanity is nicely balanced by the wonderful small shops in New York, where you can buy offbeat gifts for only a few dollars. My favourite shop is called The Elder Craftsmen. All its items are hand-made by men and women over the age of sixty. You can buy Christmas tree ornaments there that include a hand-carved wooden sledge, a pair of felt penguins, and a gnome made out of a walnut shell and wearing a bright red peaked cap. You can buy a mobile of felt figures from Beatrix Potter's Peter Rabbit stories, and another with figures from *The Nutcracker*. You can buy hand-made baby's boots and mittens, and hand-made toys, including a four-foot-long stuffed cotton dachshund.

My favourite gift came from *The New York Times*. It cost two dollars and fifty cents, and I'm giving it as a small extra present to my seven Christmas dinner guests. I found out the birth date – day, month and year – of each guest, and mailed the list of dates to a store owned by the *Times*. I got back a Xerox of the front page of *The New York Times* published on the day each guest was born. Each front page came neatly rolled like a diploma, to be wrapped and put at the guest's place, but suitable for framing later.

In spite of inflation, Christmas in New York is as lovely as ever. All the big churches are holding their usual marvellous concerts, including one at St Thomas's on Fifth Avenue, called 'An English Christmas'. But the churches, too, are feeling the pinch, and this year the concerts were no longer free.

At my house, too, things are different this Christmas – and things are also the same. My friend Nina's son Claudie, who has been coming to me for Christmas dinner since he was eleven, will be coming tomorrow in uniform – on holiday leave from the US Marine Corps. My refrigerator hasn't grown, however, so as usual my dessert is in the freezer of number 16B, and my sweet potato casserole is in the refrigerator of 4F. And though the two girls who lived up the hall in 8E are both married now, one of them still lives there, with her bridegroom; and after dinner, Richard will wheel my tea-wagon full of dishes up the hall to be put in 8E's dishwasher. Chester, his Old English sheepdog, and Duke, Nina's German shepherd who was my own true love, are both dead now. But Bentley, the abandoned sheepdog Richard adopted, is coming to dinner, and he'll trot up the hall alongside the tea-wagon as the other dogs used to.

APPLAUSE! APPLAUSE!

Kate Osborne

I went to my very last amateur theatrical event just before Christmas. It was an improvized nativity play, and although the little boy playing the innkeeper brought the house down by saying yes, he did just happen to have a room if they wouldn't mind sharing a bath, I've decided I've had enough. I don't want to see any more emaciated youths with uncertain vocal chords playing Roman generals, Renaissance cardinals, or Edwardian men about town. I don't want to sweat with apprehension watching anyone remotely connected with me waving their hands about like electrified fins, or muttering their lines into precariously attached beards. No more tinny music which doesn't start on cue, and what is worse doesn't stop when it should. No more hideous dry-ups when the only one who isn't deafened by the prompter is the person who's dried up; no more doors which refuse to open; no more swords resolutely glued to the insides of scabbards; no more false grass to send leading ladies into flying tackles. I'm through with it all.

The first show we saw as parents involved our daughter being a daffodil in an improbable choreographic display set to Tchaikovsky's *Sleeping Beauty* music. As she was very plump with glowing red cheeks, she would have been slightly more credible as a petunia or a tuber rose, but there she was, swaying about in rather a lot of bright yellow crepe paper, looking like a top-heavy toy trumpet with legs. The whole outfit looked very precarious, and as she approached the footlights and saw us she waved, fell over in her excitement, and was plucked from the chorus line by one of those long poles teachers use for opening classroom windows. As the manipulator of the pole was invisible to the audience, it was quite the most dramatic thing in the show. Despite this unfortunate debut, the following year she landed the part of Tinkerbell, and as flying wires were out of the question she had to pretend to be airborne by flitting about the stage more or less all the time. A kindly critic might have described her performance as giving a new solidity to the character, but all we heard were the alarming thumps as she threw herself enthusiastically into the part. We were greatly relieved when she started to grow upwards instead of outwards, and got jolly swaggering parts like woodmen with axes and young princes from far-off lands looking for suitable brides.

Our next daughter was more slightly built, and in her first year at secondary school came home one day with the news that she too was to be a fairy – this time the piece was *A Midsummer Night's Dream*. 'Which fairy?' I asked. 'Oh, I haven't got a name', she said carelessly. 'Fiona, Pauline and me are just general fairies.' Thank God for that, I thought. Some other hapless parent can cringe over Pease Blossom and Moth. We enjoyed the evening a lot. We smirked over other people's children being simply terrible and thought that with all that soft lighting she looked quite nice as the Fairy Chorus. Until the very end, that is, when Titania and Oberon trip away, making no stay, and all that kind of thing. As 'Fiona, Pauline and me' made their exits they managed not only to trip themselves, but also to take all the artificial trees with them. In the terrible silence that followed, the anguished voice of their English teacher could be heard from the wings: 'Useless fairies! You've ruined everything!' followed almost immediately by heart-rending sobs from the offending sprites. She never got another part. 'Her work lacks attention to detail,' said her drama report, 'and her co-ordination leaves a great deal to be desired.'

At our son's school they went through a dreadful period of improvized drama. You know the sort of thing – happenings like *A Day in the Life of an English Meadow*. His drama teacher, a young girl with leanings towards Freud, explained in the programme notes that The Drama and The Dance enabled the class to express themselves and release their tensions. The result was usually disastrous.

After that my son had nothing to do with the Thespian arts until he went to college, and then because he fancied a girl in the dramatic society he got involved in a production of *Waiting for Godot*. To our horror he asked us to go up and see it. It's not the most riveting of plays at the best of times, but after a four-hour journey, a large plate of spaghetti bolognese and rather too much wine, it was an endurance test. Wedged into a chair which had been designed by a sadist, I fell into a series of uneasy dozes, waking up each time to hear the same exchange: 'Can we go now?' 'No . . . not yet: we're waiting for Godot.' It seemed to last for hours, and by the time we left the theatre I felt almost as bad as the tramps in the play looked, and with better reason – they, after all, had been sitting in comfortable dustbins all evening.

No, I've done my stint. I never want to taste the magic of the amateur theatre again . . . never want to thrill to the smell of the greasepaint and the roar of the extras jostling about backstage. As far as I'm concerned, the show can go on for as long as it likes – for ever if necessary – just as long as I don't have to watch it!

RACE PREJUDICE

In 1972 Carol Carnall started an organization called Harmony, for multiracial families. Here she talks about her own personal experience of the kind of problems encountered

I am white and my children are mixed race, as their father came from Africa. A few years ago my six-year-old daughter, Natasha, kept bringing home the same two books from her school library. Significantly they appeared to be the only two multi-racial books that the library possessed: *Your Skin and Mine* and *The Hollywell Family*. Natasha is very aware that she's black, and she could identify with the children in those books in a way that was impossible with the remainder – books peopled with white characters.*

That same year Natasha saw a film at a local church club about leprosy in India. She arrived home anxious to talk about it. After she had been reassured that she couldn't catch leprosy from Indian families here, her first question was, 'Mum, can black people become doctors?' The doctor in the film was a white missionary. It was a shock to me that Natasha needed to ask such a question. But then I thought about it. Our own doctor was white. Had she in fact ever seen a black doctor? Yet there were many black doctors in hospitals. I checked through our children's books and we had none in which black people were shown in roles of authority.

I then went to talk to her teacher in her school, a lively multi-racial primary on the edge of south London. I explained to the young teacher that these two incidents had convinced me that Natasha's sense of herself as a black person was not being met adequately at school, and I freely admitted my former blindness to the situation at home. While we were talking I noticed a collage of faces on the wall. Natasha's class was very mixed, over half the children being black or brown, yet all the faces in the wall display were white except for a Red Indian chief. So Natasha and all the other non-white children could not point to any face at all and say, 'That's like me.'

The teacher was very uneasy talking about race, and she was uncomfortable with the term 'black'. 'You see,' she said, 'I don't discriminate at all. I make sure I treat them all the same.' And by the work on the wall and the all-white books on the shelves I realized that she meant, 'I treat all my class as if they are white', which is devastating if you happen to be black.

Last year we moved north of London to a predominantly white area, and here we found name-calling in abundance – 'wog' or 'Paki' usually; and it happened in schools where initially the teachers said, when asked about race: 'We have no problems here.' People often play down name-calling where racial insults are bandied about, saying that it's no different from being called 'fatty' or 'four eyes'. But of course being fat or wearing glasses doesn't exclude you from jobs, or incline teachers to assume that you are dim. Moreover it has nothing to do with a well-organized system of racial superiority and very real feelings of antagonism.

Natasha is nine now. A few months ago she came home from school sobbing, her fragile sense of her black self shattered. So many children were calling her 'wog' – in assembly, in class, on her way into school. We talked about it, and at one point Natasha said, 'When they say "wog" they look at me as if it was something that they didn't like for pudding, and it was disgusting.' The children who called Natasha 'wog' have probably almost no positive experience of black people, and for them the lack of multi-cultural materials at home, at school and in the media is mostly responsible for such antagonistic, racist behaviour.

Natasha has since found that replying to racial insults by retorting 'white ice cream' has effectively silenced the name-callers. A boy who called out 'wog' as he walked past Natasha was so incensed by being called a white ice cream in reply that he came back and shouted, 'Don't you ever say that again.' As he hasn't repeated his own insult, she hasn't needed to. Another boy, given the same treatment, was about to repeat the insult a little later. Just in time he remembered the earlier incident and quickly apologized.

Answering back gives the name-callers experience of being on

229

the receiving end, harmless as the phrase 'white ice cream' is. And it stops a child from feeling a helpless victim. I realize that I'm partly responsible for their ability to wound Natasha and make her shrivel up inside and say passionately to me, 'I wish they knew how it feels.' I did not consciously build up her confidence and pride in her colour in those first vital five years. And her temperament particularly needs this reinforcing approach.

Many parents have this experience, and in Harmony it has hit us hard. We cannot allow school and the community to get away with making black and brown children feel marginal or invisible. We must make our homes reflect our multi-cultural community, and part of this process involves consciously choosing books and toys that are relevant – materials that reflect both white and black in society. And I think white children may grow up with racist attitudes unless their parents introduce them to multi-racial books and toys at home. Moreover we have discovered that, if we start doing this early enough, from the moment we begin to talk to our children when they are babies, they grow up with a positive, good feeling about being black; and this feeling of self-worth is an inner strength which no one can take away.

*Harmony produces a multi-cultural children's booklist, available price 50p from 42 Beech Drive, Boreham Wood, Herts, WD6 4QU

PROFESSIONAL ETHICS

Four people in whose lives and work ethics play a large part talk about their own particular attitudes, experiences and codes of practice. First Anthony Quinton, President of Trinity College, Oxford, and formerly a Fellow of All Souls

Ethics is a slightly tiresome word because it's used in two different ways. It's used sometimes for a more or less reflective or critical activity of thinking about how people ought to think about morality, about principles of conduct. It's also used in a particular connection, where one talks about the ethics of a profession, and there it simply means the specific morality of that profession or the rules about what ought to be done that apply to members of that profession in a way they don't apply to other people.

In some circumstances what contributes to human beings' welfare will differ from what contributed in the past. To take a very simple example, the very first settlers in Australia could throw their garbage out without anybody being harmed – wallabies and kangaroos would consume it, no doubt. But nowadays empty cans of Foster's beer and so forth, if thrown out by the congested inhabitants of Sydney, would cause repulsive consequences.

Some variation is permissible within the general bounds of what is ethical, and that raises two questions. One is that people disagree about what the correct rules of conduct are, and the other is that even where everybody does agree what the rules of conduct are, they don't all live up to them. So there are two ways in which actual conduct can deviate from the ideal. Take vegetarianism, for instance – all parties can get on fine provided that the person hostile to meat-eating recognizes some limits. It is perfectly all right for him not to eat meat himself, and it's perfectly all right for him to talk in a persuasive manner to other people, to make his case as energetically as he can against meat-eating; but if he starts leading riotous mobs of principled vegetarians in assaults on butchers we are confronted with a difficult social problem.

The trouble, clearly, is that an awful lot of people are not satisfied to be virtuous themselves, and find it intolerable to think that other people aren't virtuous – and this isn't always a terribly virtuous impulse, if I may put it so. It doesn't seem to me a field in which one can be as certain as people are traditionally supposed to be. To put it very simply, there was a theologian, once much studied, called Archdeacon Paley, who said something like this. It's perfectly evident that the way in which we find out what we ought to do is by consulting what will most contribute to human happiness, because we know that God is concerned with the happiness of His creatures. He wants them to act so that they shall in general be happy. Therefore, to find out what God wants us to do, we find out what will, in general, contribute to human happiness. This doesn't mean what contributes to each individual's happiness at the expense of others, but what is the overall way of maximizing happiness. And that is something that is hard to work out in many cases, something it is often unreasonable to be certain about.

When one first reflects on the human phenomenon of morality, one considers that it consists largely of rules of universal application. I oughtn't to steal, you oughtn't to steal, nobody else ought to steal. It applies to all of us. But there are some rules that apply, we feel, specifically to some individuals and not to others. For instance, I have a special responsibility to my children which other people in general, apart from my wife, don't have, and that's incumbent on me because of a special situation in which I am. Then I have some other duties because I've made promises or undertakings of some sort or another.

It seems to me that the ethics of a profession is really an extended case of a duty or a responsibility arising from an undertaking or commitment. Sometimes this is more or less explicit. The newly recruited soldier takes an oath of allegiance to the Queen, which I daresay embodies some readiness to accept the lawful authority of sergeants. In the field of medicine, doctors take the Hippocratic oath, which defines certain special responsibilities that are incumbent on doctors because of the particular relationships to human beings in which they find themselves. People may say that a profession will generate an ethic of its own for its own professional welfare, and of course in a way it does – at least a profession will tend to police its own ethics, which is to some extent advantageous to it, because it's better that it should do so for itself than that other perhaps less sympathetic persons should do so for it. I think people often worry about this when, for instance, the rights and wrongs of the incompetence of lawyers are decided upon by other lawyers. It applies particularly to lawyers, of course, because it's people who are or have been lawyers who have a very focal position in tribunals and bodies making judgements of one sort or another. When people complain about medical treatment it may come before some medical body, but in the end it's a matter for the law. But at any rate, in any profession there will tend to be a recognition of specific responsibilities incumbent on the members of that profession.

Ann Mallalieu, a barrister and former President of the Cambridge Union, on ethics at the bar

Lawyers' ethics are set out in a little book on etiquette which every barrister is given on the night that he is called by his inn – the night he really starts practice. It consists basically of commonsense decisions and rulings that have been made by the Bar Council over the years, as various problems have arisen. But in addition to that there is an over-riding unwritten code concerning the way you behave in cases and the way you behave in connection with your client and other barristers. Every barrister learns this at his pupil master's knee – in other words, when he goes around during the early stages with a senior barrister, watching how things are done, before he's allowed to practise.

As a lawyer, one is in the unique position of being exclusively concerned with right and wrong. However if every time one picked up a brief one thought of the morality of what one was doing, and the morality of what one's client had or had not done, that would cause one to overlook the real reason for the barrister's presence, which is not to judge anybody in any way, or to take a particular moral stance, but to present the case that has been given to one to the best of one's ability as an advocate.

All barristers are on a kind of cab rank. One occasionally hears people say that they never prosecute, but that is in fact contrary to the ethics of the bar. If you practise in a particular field, and you're free to do so, then you are supposed to accept the solicitor's instructions.

As regards one's moral obligations to accept a case, there is a very strict code. If a defendant tells a barrister that he committed the offence in question but wants to plead not guilty, the barrister must say that he has a duty not only to the client but also to the court, because he has been called to the bar: it's a double duty. No barrister is allowed to put in court, to a witness, anything which he knows to be untrue. If the defendant insists on pleading not guilty, even though he tells the barrister that he is in fact guilty, his counsel can ask no witness any question, nor can he say anything to the judge or to the jury, which he knows is wrong. As a result, the defending counsel would be fighting his client's case with his hands tied behind his back. He should advise the defendant to go to another barrister.

If a barrister is prosecuting against an inexperienced defence counsel, it puts him in a slightly odd position which is something that people outside the profession find mystifying. Obviously, whether you're prosecuting or defending, your job is to present the case as clearly and as fairly as you can. But if you're prosecuting and someone on the other side misses what you think is an important point there are two responses to the situation. If defence counsel is experienced and ought to know better, on the whole that's bad luck for him, but if it's someone who is not as experienced as they might be, or who has overlooked something important that day, nine times out of ten the prosecuting counsel will come and say something like: 'Have you seen this case? Have a look at that paragraph of Archbold, and you may get some idea there.' I remember when I first started at the bar, just before I got up to cross-examine a witness, the prosecutor leaned over and showed me another statement which that witness had made, but which I'd not been given. It gave a different version of the story, and was of great assistance to me. That is really where the second duty of the prosecuting counsel comes in. His job is not simply to put the case for the prosecution evidence; he also has a duty to the court to try and get at the truth of the matter.

Of course it's the client who often suffers if his counsel has missed a point, which many people find a little strange in a profession which is concerned with justice. The judge, however, is supposed to be keeping the balance in court. The way in which the case is conducted undoubtedly does determine the kind of situation in which a particular prosecutor finds himself – often in some embarrassment if he has to correct or remind someone more senior than himself on the other side. At the end of the day, of course, it is the judge who is supposed to be seeing fair play and making sure that all the defences are put properly to the jury.

Some people wonder if a barrister finds it hard, when he first meets a client, not to form an instinctive judgement about his guilt, and if he does, to be quite sure that it is eliminated from his presentation of the client's case. I don't try to eliminate this assessment from my decision on how the client should approach the case. When I see him beforehand, in order to advise him I must go into the case with open eyes, and look at it plainly, possibly even forming some view on the evidence I've got. When I get into court I'm not doing my job for my client if in the back of my mind I'm thinking, 'My goodness! It all depends on me whether this innocent man goes away or not. I must put everything into it.' As soon as I have that extra pressure on me of, for example, believing firmly that the man is innocent and shouldn't be in the dock, and then allow that to dominate my thinking, I don't plead the case as well as I should, because I don't see the different issues, and I don't see the points as clearly as I should if

I were dispassionate. In many ways it's much easier to defend somebody whom you believe in the back of your mind to be guilty, but who insists on fighting the case, than it is to defend someone whom you think is probably not guilty and who is fighting it.

For these reasons I think that clarity of mind is perhaps a more useful quality in a barrister than compassion. When you're conducting a case compassion obviously takes different forms. I think it's important to be able to understand the feelings of your client in order to be able to communicate them by your defence to the jury. And I think that a barrister who can eliminate human feeling and motivation won't be doing the best for his client, because he might well be presenting the case in a way which made it less acceptable to, and understandable by, the jury. But the old days of the criminal advocates who used to burst into tears and shout and declaim and wave at the jury have gone. I think it's because jurors now tend to be far more intelligent and sophisticated, better able to look at the facts of the case, and therefore less swayed by the advocacy or histrionics of the person presenting the case. I must admit, though, to thinking that court rooms must have been tremendous places in those days. When you read through the whole speeches of people like Marshall Hall you can see how stirring it must have been to observe those wonderful, old-hat tricks of allowing time to elapse in total silence and then producing tears, literally tears, which you would never see in a court today.

James Anderton, Chief Constable of Greater Manchester, explains how his personal moral attitudes influence his approach to law enforcement

I come from a very Christian family, one that has always been committed to public service, and it seemed to me that being a policeman would enable me to carry through into my professional life the deep personal convictions I hold. At one stage the minister of my church, with whom I had a very close affinity because my family was heavily involved in local church work, suggested that I might consider the Church as a career – a calling if you like, which is really what it is – and I thought about it. I taught in Sunday school, as did my wife, whom I was courting at the time, but eventually I decided against it. I don't know whether I made the right decision or not. Some people very unkindly say that it was a toss-up whether I became a police officer or a preacher, and my enemies say it's a pity I lost the toss! At this time my wife also converted me to Methodism. I was brought up in the Church of England, although historically my family was one of the strongest Roman Catholic families in the north-west, but when I met my wife she was such a delightful person that I couldn't refuse anything she asked of me, and I simply converted myself to Methodism.

I certainly feel I have had more influence where I am than I would if I had gone into the Church. One of the things I have complained about quite vociferously in recent years is the apparent ineptitude of the Church, or Churches, and their leaders. I felt that they ought to have been standing up more often in public, speaking out about the things that were clearly wrong and needed to be put right. But instead they have embarked upon all kinds of political travels and journeys, and not attended to the very things that the public and their people wanted them to do. If I had been in that position, I might have been caught up in the same way. Now, as a chief constable, and without wishing to misuse or abuse my powers and privileged position, I can do all of those things. I can speak with a very public voice about matters concerning the public at large within my own province; I can also express my deep moral convictions; and I can make what some regard as political comments about the things that are going wrong within society as a whole.

I believe that human nature contains something very elementary. Most people distinguish clearly between right and wrong, and know that difference from the time that they are very young children. People know what it is within human nature that has to be controlled, regulated and corrected. They know what it is within society that demands of us all, in a community sense, a caring and compassionate disposition, and all of this is embraced by the term 'fundamental moralist'. If I am described as such, I hope that I am not regarded in any sense as a bigot or somebody who closes his mind to changing circumstances and conditions, because society and human nature do change to a certain extent according to the influences that are currently brought to bear upon them, and that has to be taken account of, too.

As a policeman, of course, I don't find it as simple as all this may sound, because there can be conflict between doing what one thinks is right, and one's responsibility to uphold the law. The great problem with the law is that it is not absolute or finite. The law can do anything: it promoted slavery in America, it supports apartheid in South Africa, and in Germany before and during the Second World War it enabled people to attempt the genocide of the Jews. You cannot simply say 'the law', and leave it at that. You have to be satisfied in your heart that the law is humane, just and equitable, and that it is properly and lawfully enforced, too. You can have good law badly enforced as much as you can have bad law which ought not to exist in the first place.

Some people in Greater Manchester, referring to my campaign against pornography and obscenity, have suggested that I am out of tune with reality. They have argued that I am trying to impose upon people with twentieth-century ideas a kind of eighteenth-century moralism, and I disagree entirely with that. I enforce the law in that particular area with due discretion, mostly as a result of public complaints to me, and exercising my own judgement as a police officer. I am not, I suspect, out of touch with reality at all. In fact I feel that within the community as a whole, and certainly in my own area of Greater Manchester, there is a great reawakening of community spirit, a great sense within people that they want to see a return to the standards and values and concepts of righteousness that used to exist, and upon which people could found their lives.

A police officer's responsibilities are widely spread, because he has to be sensitive to the needs of the whole community. He has to be concerned about the victim of a crime as he is about the person who commits it. A policeman cannot simply look at the situation and imagine that he can deal with one part of it and ignore the effect upon everybody else at the same time. He has to be conscious of his responsibility to the law-abiding community, he has to be sympathetic and caring towards the victims of crimes, and necessarily he has to be very conscious of what it is that has brought an offender into the realm of criminal activity and indeed into police hands and in front of the court.

The police force has a rigid discipline and a distinct hierarchy, and some people have suggested that a chief constable has more power than is desirable. It certainly may seem from time to time that we are all-powerful, and in an operational sense we are, because we have very considerable freedom in that respect, but that is a freedom under the law, which places its own constraints upon us. We also take great account of the opinions and views of Parliament and the Home Secretary, and we would be very foolish indeed if we did not.

That of course is talking about ultimate accountability; in the immediate sense, however, one is accountable to oneself. I have to impose on myself the discipline that comes from the knowledge that, as a president of the United States once said, 'The buck stops here.' I am like a goldfish in a bowl – everybody sees me for what I am and what I do, and that is part of my personal means of accounting to the public. If I speak out, if I tell people not only what I am and who I am but why I do things, that is the greatest possible safeguard for the people with whom I have to deal. I don't hide anything from myself, my officers or the public. I am very much a believer in open accounting, in explaining myself to the public as often as I can.

Television reporter Richard Lindley

I like to work both at home and abroad. I feel that, if you don't stay in touch with what people are thinking and feeling at home, it's very difficult to do your job properly. I notice that permanent foreign correspondents abroad sometimes just miss the questions that people at home want to have asked on their behalf.

Some people think that the truth is sometimes too horrible to reveal to the public, but on the whole I feel it's unethical not to do so. The only time I've been really angry with my immediate employers, the television company, was when I was in Vietnam, as I was on a number of occasions. Every day we'd go down the road to try and cover the war, and we'd aim to get a sense of what war was like. That's why I was there: to report the war as it actually was. One day we fell upon a particularly bloody incident which we were also able to cover. Normally you can't do both – either it's a very bloody piece of war which you can't film for practical reasons, or else it's not very exciting. This time it was remarkable and horrific – a close encounter with grenades being thrown, and people being blown in the air and killed. At the end we had some pretty gruesome film, but it showed what had happened that day. I got a message back from the office saying, 'Wonderful film. Of course we couldn't use the close-ups.' That seemed to me to be cheating – we had recorded what the war was like, but the company had transmitted a sanitized version of that truth.

I think I was concerned most of all that the camera crew and I had risked our lives, and our material hadn't been on the screen in the way that it ought to have been. We'd had a particularly sweaty time, so that's purely selfish, but I have to be honest and admit that that was my first reaction. Secondly, I think the public was being cheated. People watching that programme just weren't being told the truth.

I believe that reporters perhaps cheat a little, though, in different ways. Our role of coming in, observing, listening, asking questions, and then going away and making a report enables us sometimes to use that as an excuse for not being involved. It's very convenient to say, 'I'm sorry, I have to stand back from this and try to decide what's going on here and tell other people about it. That's my role and nothing else.' But one does feel very responsible for ensuring that significant or important points of view are put. I got very angry a couple of years ago when there seemed to be a sort of liberal conspiracy to deny racial feeling in Britain. Perfectly understandably, for the best of liberal reasons, the broadcasting organizations and the newspapers felt that it was not helpful, for example, to let the white residents of a particularly unpleasant block of flats in inner London, who were having a very hard time from a large number of black immigrants, moan and complain and be insulting in public. That seemed to me wrong. The pressures were very great indeed, but I felt that even if it was being done for the right reasons it was quite wrong to suppress that point of view. You had to let it be expressed; you had to question it; you had to ask people whether they were being racist or whether they were being factual and sensible and practical. That point of view had to be heard, and eventually it did get heard.

There are occasions, of course, when you've just got to stop doing your job and attend to something more pressing. If somebody is wounded at your side in a war situation – which doesn't, frankly, happen very often – you do something about it, and that must come first. But the job of the reporter is primarily to show what goes on, and if possible not to stop, but to carry on and let people understand what the situation really is. I did stop once though, in Dacca, now the capital of Bangladesh but then still in East Pakistan. At the end of the war between India and Pakistan over that patch of territory the guerilla leader was haranguing a large number of his victorious warriors in the stadium in Dacca, and below the platform were a pathetic group of some twenty captured prisoners. Every time he shouted, the people down below would prod these wretched men with bayonets, and kick them and generally abuse them. We filmed a little of this – there was another television team there, too – and then became increasingly worried that our presence there was encouraging them to torture these people. So we started putting our cameras down and sitting on them. But it still went on, and we became convinced that perhaps the situation was caused by our very presence there. It got very, very unpleasant indeed and both camera crews almost simultaneously felt that we could not remain there, so we left.

Hardly had we arrived back at the hotel than a couple of still photographer colleagues who had stayed there came rushing back, saying that the prisoners had in fact been butchered before their very eyes. Bayonets had been thrust into them and they had been killed in the most barbarous and bloody way. The two photographers won a Pulitzer prize for their pictures, and we got questions from our offices – polite but concerned – as to why we hadn't been there and why we hadn't filmed. I'm still not really sure whether we should have stayed or whether we were right to have left.

Sometimes demonstrations are organized with the sole purpose of being reported on television, and the increasing sophistication of modern equipment makes us constantly conscious of the ethical problems involved. We have the ability to eavesdrop on people's conversations with directional microphones. Should we wire people up with microphones so that they can conduct interviews with people who don't know that they're being interviewed? But I think the issues basically remain the same: you have to decide whether you're going to do that or not.

I'm very suspicious of the idea of objectivity in my work. I think it's quite right that, for example, the BBC has distinguished in the past between news and current affairs, though I think that now, perhaps, the two should come together. The idea is that in my sort of work, current affairs, you spend long enough on a subject to get some idea of what you think about it. The public's protection against having just one view foisted on it is that there are always a number of views on any subject. I remember something the head of my department said when there was a row over a film I'd made about Iran, in which I'd said that the Shah was ordering too many British tanks for his own good and our good. The Foreign Office was a bit upset about that, but his answer to me was, 'I pay you to go and make up your mind.' That seems to me to be the only basis on which one can work.

CUSTARD TART

Mary Berry's recipe serves four to six

Pastry
4 oz (125 g) plain flour
1½ oz (40 g) butter
1 oz (30 g) lard
1 egg yolk
½ oz (15 g) caster sugar
about 1 teaspoon cold water

Custard
2 eggs
1 oz (30 g) caster sugar
½ pint (300 ml) milk
a little grated nutmeg

First make the pastry. Put the flour in a bowl, add the fats cut in small pieces, and rub in with your fingertips until the mixture resembles fine breadcrumbs. Mix the egg yolk with the sugar and water, and stir into the dry ingredients to bind them together. Roll out the pastry on a floured surface. Place in a 7 inch (18 cm) greased flan ring on a greased baking sheet and chill for 30 minutes. Pre-heat the oven to 425°F (220°C, gas mark 7). Line the pastry with foil or greaseproof paper, weigh down with empty smaller tins or baking beans, and bake blind for 15 minutes.

Meanwhile prepare the custard. Beat the eggs and sugar together until blended and then stir in the milk. Remove the foil or greaseproof paper, and tins or beans, from the flan. Reduce the oven temperature to 400°F (200°C, gas mark 6). Pour the custard mixture into the flan and sprinkle with a little grated nutmeg. Bake for 15 minutes, then reduce the heat again and cook for a further 25 minutes at 350°F (180°C, gas mark 4), or until the filling is set and a pale golden brown. Serve warm on the day it is made.

UP THE CROSSING*

Ken Ausden

Many's the day I've been up the crossing and seen five Castles and three Kings in the space of not much more than half an hour. Not to mention the Halls, the Courts, the Manors, the Bulldogs and the vast assortment of unnamed goods engines, like the 2-6-os, the pannier tanks and the hulking great 2-8-o Consolidations. Like my Gramp used to say, 'Anybody that's never seen the Cheltenham Flyer come leapin' an' roarin' under the first bridge – that's never been wrapped in a grey-black shawl of engine smoke – that's never seen a double-header snortin' an' slippin' at the signal tryin' to take off wi' a 'undred an' more wagons – they've missed some o' the joy in life.'

I reckon he was dead right, too. How can you get excited about a diesel electric? As hygienic as a plastic bag and about as interesting. The sort of engine you could drive wearing your Sunday suit.

I feel sorry for the kids today – I mean, not being able to go up the crossing like we used to do and breathe nothing but choking smoke and warm steam and oil smells all day long. Those school holidays in 1938 were something special.

We would set off about ten in the morning with a day's supply of fish-paste sandwiches and our engine-name books and stubs of pencil pinched from school. Georgie carried his rations in a brown paper carrier bag; Albie had his sister's tatty old school satchel slung round his neck; Spud's food would be wrapped in a sheet of greaseproof paper and tied up with string, and he always carried it stuffed up his jersey so he had his hands free for emergencies; I lugged along a battered, fraying attaché case which I had found in my Dad's allotment shed and which was secured with a red-and-white-striped trouser belt because the rusted lock had long since given up functioning.

But the envy of us all was Vic. He always led the way – I can see him now, his Gran-knitted grey socks slipping down his calves as he strode out ahead of the rest of us. We would shuffle along a few paces behind him, our eyes taking in every detail of the passing scene, yet always coming back to rest enviously on the brown canvas bag swinging so proudly from Vic's shoulder.

For that bag had travelled on more trains than any of us had seen sunrises. It had belonged to Vic's Gramp. And Vic's Gramp had been a top link guard. He'd risen from being a shunter down the con yard, first to a goods guard and then a passenger guard. He had been on duty on six Royal Trains and had actually shaken hands with the King. I wondered what the King thought of Vic's Gramp's bag!

I'd seen plenty of guards on their way to and from the junction station with their bags slung from their shoulders, their red and green flags poking out from under the flaps. Actually to own a real guard's bag like Vic had – to have a Gramp who had travelled on all the top express trains all over the GWR – it wasn't fair really! And my Gramp only a boiler-maker!

Vic's bag looked as old as his Gramp. It had a genuine oil stain on one side and some different-coloured stitching where Vic's Gran had repaired the shoulder strap many times. It was faded and creased and greasy and altogether a most beautiful bag, a genuine railwayman's bag. Vic's sandwiches even tasted better than ours, as if the very smoke and steam and oil and coal dust of forty years had seeped into the bread itself.

It was a two-mile trek to the crossing along a main road. But once we got to the slaughterhouse and climbed the fence into the field that led to the railway track, the world of streets and pavements, petrol-driven cars and horse-drawn carts, houses and schools, parents and teachers and all the other trivia of life was put behind us. Ahead lay the gleaming tracks, parallel pairs of dull metal rails polished to a sparkling silver by a million speeding wheels.

'Come on!' Vic would yell the second we were over the fence and in sight of the engines. 'Let's get a good place on the bank afore the Chapel Street gang gets 'ere.'

We raced for the gently sloping cutting close to the main up line.

'We'll jus' be in time for the 10.36 Pad', puffed Spud, his fat legs scuttling through the mowing grass. As if in answer, a distant whistle from the junction station signalled the departure of the 10.36 non-stop express train to Paddington.

'Bet it's *Windsor Castle* pullin' it', chirruped Albie.

'Bet yer a pound', I said.

'You mus' know somethin' if yer bettin' more money than you've ever owned', said Vic.

'How d'you know it won't be *Windsor Castle*?' asked Albie.

' 'Cos she's been in the sheds for repairs all week an' she ain't done a trial run yet', I announced proudly. (Having a Gramp who was a boiler-maker could be useful sometimes!)

'I reckon it'll be *Berry Pomeroy*', said Georgie.

'If I've seen *Berry Pomeroy* once I've seen 'er an 'undred times', moaned Albie. 'I 'ope it's one I ain't seen afore.'

'I've seen all the Castle class', I said, swanking. 'I'm seein' most Castles for the 'undredth time.'

We snuggled down in the long grass only a few feet from the up main – near enough almost to feel the power and energy of the great driving wheels as *Berry Pomeroy* and twelve coaches roared by, building up speed for her seventy-seven-mile journey to London.

We lay in our nest in the grass for a couple of hours, watching express trains and milkies and goods and shunting engines adding their contributions of noise and smell and excitement to the joy of a holiday morning, and occasionally enjoying a bit of a scrap among ourselves to keep the blood moving.

'Hey, there!'

A voice, distant yet urgent. A grown-up, man's voice, the sort that sets small boys running away without stopping to ask what they've done wrong. We crouched low in our hide-out. My mind ran expertly through the possibilities. The farmer because we'd trodden down his mowing grass? A railway copper because we were trespassing? The shopkeeper from down the road where Vic had put a ha'penny in the Beechnut chewing-gum machine and thumped it with his fist to try and make two packets come out at one pull?

'Hey there, you kids!'

The voice sounded more imploring than angry now – like my Dad when he wanted me to run over the Co-op and get him twenty cork-tipped.

I peered over the grassy parapet like an infantryman weighing up the enemy position. A fat man in an apron and a straw boater was standing over the far side of the field, waving his arms and hollering.

'What's up wi' 'im?' muttered Vic, close to my left ear.

'Dunno', I answered. 'Looks as if 'e's 'avin' a fit!'

Then we saw the other occupant of the field. A black and white dappled horse was prancing through the long grass, heading straight for the crossing. 'Stop 'im! Stop 'im!' yelled the distant fat man. 'E'll kill 'isself!'

Kill 'isself he certainly would if he trotted on to the permanent way with about four expresses and any number of goods trains due along in the next few minutes.

Vic, who was supposed to lead our gang, made no move. Nor did any of the others. They were probably thinking. Very slowly. But this was a time for action, not thoughts. Or perhaps I was the only one who wasn't too scared of horses. Anyway, I upped and dashed along the embankment towards the spot where the horse looked as though it would career on to the tracks. I began yelling, just any old things that came into my head.

'Whoa! Get back! Stupid animal!'

The horse ignored me. I tried to run faster, but the long grass imprisoned my legs. I yelled louder and waved my arms around like a small, mobile windmill. The horse cantered steadily on, looking neither to right nor to left. It must have been about fifty yards from the crossing when I saw the banner of white smoke signalling the fast up-milk. I slithered down the embankment on to the rough ballast and began running along the sleepers – the bits that stuck out at the side of the rails. I saw the horse teetering on the brink of the downward slope, pawing the long grass to find a footing. A quick glance ahead at the round, black blob of approaching engine with its halo of smoke and steam, and I was off the sleepers and dashing towards the bank. The horse was tipped forward at a crazy angle as it gingerly felt its way down.

'Get back, boy! Whoa, there!' My voice had to compete with

the clanking and chuffing of the 4-6-o loco. 'Wait there, boy! I'm coming!'

I picked up a handful of ballast and hurled it at the horse's front legs. It spattered in the grass and he hesitated. Another handful smacked him in the chest and he backed up a pace or two. The up-milk let out a fearful shriek as it clattered past, though whether the whistling was a sign of anger towards a small boy on the line or of warning to the horse, I shall never know. Anyway, the horse, suddenly petrified by the din of the rumbling milk wagons, stood his ground. Before I had to make the momentous decision whether to try to catch him by his bridle, cowboy fashion, the fat man arrived and did it for me. . . .

'Never know 'im do nothin' like it, not in all the six years I've 'ad 'im', the fat man confided, taking off his straw hat to wipe the globs of sweat from his forehead. 'The times I've let 'im out o' the shafts in that very spot so's 'e could 'ave a stretch an' a bite o fresh grass. Dunno what got into 'im today, I don't.'

But I wasn't listening to him particularly. I was enjoying every bounding moment of my first-ever ride on the driver's seat of a delivery cart: *Johnson's Fresh Fish Delivered to your Door Daily*.

'D'you want a ride?' the fat man had asked me when we got the horse safely re-attached to his cart.

I was too overcome to reply. I just put one foot on the iron step and was up on the seat in a flash. Vic and Albie and the rest of 'em watched wide-eyed with envy, as I rode off like the Lord Mayor in his coach. They were welcome to their engines today. I had moved into the world of horses.

'You want to drive?' the fat man said, quite casually, as if he was asking me if I liked liquorice.

'Me! Drive!'

' 'Ere!' He handed me the reins. 'Don't choke 'im', he added as I gripped the leather straps like a drowning man clutching at straws. 'Just a touch to make 'im go right an' left an' a flick to make 'im shift 'isself, tha's all!'

I drove that horse and cart right through the centre of town, sitting up there like Lord Muck, erect and proud outside and trembling with fear inside. Right down Fleet Street and Farringdon Road we went, in and out of lorries and vans and bikes, with me in charge and my travelling companion exchanging greetings with all the bread-van drivers and milk-float pushers and Walls' ice-cream tricycle-men.

'Why don't you get yourself a decent 'orse?' he yelled at the Co-op delivery man. 'That thing o' yourn looks as if he died a fortnight ago!'

'Morning, officer', he greeted the policeman by the Town Hall, touching his straw hat in a mock salute.

'Mornin', Wally', answered the constable. 'Who's the whipper-snapper, then?'

I bent low over the reins for fear he should recognize the whipper-snapper as one of the criminals he had chased along the canal towpath a few days back for riding three on a bike!

'What d'you think o' this little feller-me lad, eh?' said Wally to the other men in Johnson's Fish Emporium when we drove into the yard. 'Saved our Snowball 'ere from bein' churned into cats' meat by the up-milk, 'e did.' He gave Snowball a sledgehammer pat with one huge, red, fishy hand while lifting me down from my perch with the other. 'What we gonna give 'im, then, for a reward? The fishmonger's Victoria Cross?'

He chortled happily away while we put Snowball in his box and then he led me to his office at the back of the shop.

'What d'you think o' that, then?'

He threw open the door and stood back to watch my face. My eyes nearly popped out of my head. I don't quite know what I expected to see, but I certainly didn't think it would be a railway museum. The walls were covered with photos of engines and old time-tables and posters advertising holidays at faraway GWR places like Newquay and Teignmouth and Tenby. There were books about railways scattered over the desk and piled up in the corners of the room. On the mantelpiece was a model of *King George V*, perfect scale, about two feet long.

'Jus' 'cos I drive a fish-cart don't mean I don't know nothin' about engines', he said, shoving me into the room. 'I was train-spottin' up the crossin', where you was this mornin', years afore you was ever thought of.'

'Who made that?' I breathed, unable to take my eyes off the miniature *King George V*.

'My Dad', said Wally, proudly. 'An' not only did 'e make it, 'e drove it. The real one, I mean.'

'Your Dad drove *King George V*?' I gasped, all incredulous. Fancy me talking to a man whose Dad drove the immortal *King!*

'Dozens o' times. Prob'ly 'undreds, in fact. Till 'e retired jus' last year.'

I dragged my eyes away from it and inspected the rest of this Aladdin's cave.

'What d'you fancy then?' asked Wally, settling himself on the corner of the huge wooden desk. ' 'Cept *King George*, o' course. I wouldn't trade 'im for a hundred Snowballs.'

My gaze had settled on another object, lying in the corner almost buried under a pile of railway magazines. It was dusty and dented – and utterly desirable.

'Could I – I mean, would you?' Unable to ask for it in so many words, I pointed at the black tin box.

'You know a good 'un when you sees it.' Wally tossed the pile of magazines to the floor and swung the metal box up on to the table. 'That's 'is actual box – me Dad's I mean. Seen a few footplates, 'as that one. I dunno 'ow I'm going to part with it, but seein' as 'ow I said you could pick what you fancied. . . .'

I honestly reckon there was a tear in his eye as Wally handed over my prize. Looking back, I don't know whether I should have accepted it – but I did.

Next morning, the gang were knocking at our back door before I'd half finished my Shredded Wheat, wanting to know how I'd got on driving the horse and cart yesterday. They all had their paraphernalia ready for another day up the crossing. Albie with his satchel round his neck – Georgie lugging his brown paper carrier bag – Spud with a lump of sandwiches up his jersey – and Vic, of course, standing there swanking with his Gramp's bag slung on his shoulder.

'Shan't be a jiff', I yelled from the back scullery. 'Jus' packin' me grub.'

' 'Aven't the bottom fell out o' that ole attaché case yet?' chortled Vic. 'You'll 'ave to find summat else to carry your grub in soon.'

'I 'ave!' I said, stepping out of the back door with more swank in my little finger than Vic had in all his scrawny body.

They fell back against the coal bunker, goggle-eyed.

'It ain't – not – not a real one, like?' breathed Spud.

'It couldn't be', muttered Albie, running his hand over the metal lid. 'Could it?'

Vic knew the real thing when he saw it, though. It took him

about a minute to get over the shock, then he sidled up to me – he was a nice kid, really, was Vic. 'Who did it b'long to?' he asked.

The others crowded in to hear.

'The driver of *King George V.*'

'It never did!'

'Honest! Cross me 'eart.'

I licked my index finger and made a solemn cross over the left side of my chest. There was no arguing against that in our gang.

'I'll let you 'ave a taste o' me sandwiches later on', I said magnanimously. 'I took me chips up to bed in it las' night. They 'ad a real footplate taste to 'em!'

From then on I walked in front, swinging my driver's lunch box for all the world to see. Vic shuffled along behind, his Gramp's bag hanging limply from his shoulder.

*This story, from a collection of short stories by the same title, was read as a serial on *Woman's Hour*. For publication details see page 255

BUTTER SHORTBREAD

Mary Berry's recipe makes 16 pieces

6 oz (175 g) plain flour
3 oz (90 g) cornflour
6 oz (175 g) butter
3 oz (90 g) caster sugar

Pre-heat the oven to 325°F (180°C, gas mark 3). Sift the two flours together. In a separate large bowl cream the butter until soft. Add the sugar and beat until light and fluffy. Work in the flour mixture and then knead well together. Press out the shortbread into a shallow, greased baking tin 11 × 7 ins (28 × 18 cm), flattening the dough with your knuckles. Prick well with a fork, and cut into 16 finger shapes with a knife. Chill in the refrigerator for 15 minutes, then bake for about 35 minutes or until a very pale golden brown. Dust with caster sugar. Leave to cool in the tin for 15 minutes, then cut through again where the shortbread is marked. Lift on to a wire rack to finish cooling.

BENTLEY'S NEW YEAR'S EVE PARTY

Helene Hanff

My friend Arlene is not a dog lover, which is the least of the differences that make us the world's unlikeliest best friends. To begin with, she's twenty years younger than I. To continue, she's been twice married and divorced, while I've been single all my life.

Like me, she lives alone at present. But I live alone in a studio apartment, consisting of a living-room with functional modern furniture, and a small alcove for my desk, typewriter-table and bookshelves. Arlene lives alone in an eight-room penthouse, with a bedroom suitably decorated for Marie Antoinette, and a living-room positively alive with silver and china ornaments and glittering chandeliers.

To round out the picture, I am plain and mousy, while Arlene is black-haired, flamboyantly beautiful, and the last word in high-fashion chic. But we're the same size. And since Arlene wouldn't dream of wearing the same wardrobe two years running, she gives me her designer suits at the end of each year and I wear them for the next eight. Her apartment-house is up at the far end of my block, but Arlene has always led a high-powered social life – and in the years when I sat out on the front step with my friends Nina and Richard and their two dogs, Duke, the German shepherd, and Chester, the Old English sheepdog, Arlene never saw me there. When I tried to tell her about Duke and Chester and their canine friends, she always cut in firmly with: 'I don't want to hear about your dogs.'

But through me, Arlene did become friends with Nina and Richard. And when she and they came to my house for dinner at Thanksgiving and Christmas, Arlene was resigned to having Duke and Chester as her fellow dinner-guests. When both dogs died, two years ago, she was genuinely distressed for our sake, but she didn't exactly miss them. And so, last Thanksgiving, Richard called me early in the day. Should he bring Bentley to dinner? 'Of course you're bringing Bentley to dinner!' I said. I hadn't told Arlene about Bentley, the abandoned Old English sheepdog Richard had adopted. But he was coming to Thanksgiving dinner, and Arlene would just have to accept him.

That evening Bentley – a huge, snowy mop of a dog – was at the door to greet Arlene, when she arrived wearing a flame-coloured, shimmering blouse and high black storm-trooper's boots with six-inch heels. While Richard made the drinks, I was busy passing hors d'oeuvres and checking on everything in the kitchen, so it was some time before I settled with my drink and glanced at Arlene. She was sitting on the sofa, with Bentley at her feet sitting with his back to her, and his head locked in a vice between her high black storm-trooper's boots. As Richard and I stared at her, Arlene yanked Bentley's head back, peered down into his eyes – one brown, one blue – and informed him: 'I like you. You're a very sophisticated dog.'

Bentley was clearly ecstatic at the mauling, but I said: 'Bite her, Bentley', whereupon Arlene pulled his head back further, prised his jaws open and stuck her fist in his mouth.

'No dog has ever crossed the threshold of my penthouse', she told him. 'But you're special. You're coming to my New Year's Eve party.'

A week later, invitations went out to fifty people – and one dog – to a New Year's Eve breakfast at Arlene's, to begin at 2.30 and run till sunrise on New Year's Day. Richard went early, to help Arlene, so Bentley – wearing a formal black bow tie – was on hand to greet the first guests. Since he took up the entire foyer, the guests

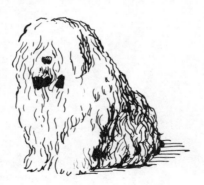

couldn't move beyond the front door till Bentley led them into the living-room, which he did. Between arrivals, Bentley circulated, sitting with first one group and then another. Now and then going to the bar to refresh himself at the sterling silver water bowl Arlene had set down for him on the floor next to the champagne bucket.

I also went to the party – kicking and screaming – having been hounded by my hostess into staying up for it. I left at quarter to four and went home to bed. Bentley had to see every departing guest to the door, so he didn't get home till 8 a.m. and spent the next two days sleeping it off. So, of course, did Arlene, and it wasn't till the third day that we hung on the phone discussing the party.

'People have been phoning all day', she said. 'Would you like to know what they talked about? Never mind the gorgeous buffet and the champagne. Never mind the great piano player. Forget I looked sensational! All anybody talked about was Bentley. Will you tell me how I can be bananas over a dog who upstaged me at my own party?'

RECIPES

BOOKS

A. J. Wentworth, BA by H. F. Ellis, published by Weidenfeld and Nicolson. Read by Arthur Lowe.

Albert and the Liner by Keith Waterhouse, published by Michael Joseph. Read by George Layton.

Blood and Judgement by Michael Gilbert, published by Hamlyn. Read by Edward Kelsey.

Close to Home by Deborah Moggach, published by Collins/Coronet. Read by Frances Jeater.

A Comfort of Cats by Doreen Tovey, published by Michael Joseph. Read by Avril Elgar.

Cousin Phillis by Elizabeth Gaskell, published by Penguin. Read by Michael Jayston.

The Crimson Chalice by Victor Canning, published by Heinemann/Penguin. Read by Martin Jarvis.

The Day of the Triffids by John Wyndham, published by Hutchinson/Penguin. Read by David Ashford.

A Death Out of Season by Emanuel Litvinoff, published by Penguin. Read by John Bennett.

The End of the Affair by Graham Greene, published by Bodley Head/Heinemann/Penguin. Read by Sian Thomas.

A Forgotten Season by Kathleen Conlon, published by Collins/Hamlyn. Read by Patricia Routledge.

A Friend of Mary Rose by Elizabeth Fenwick, published by Gollancz. Read by William Roberts.

A Glass of Blessings by Barbara Pym, published by Cape/Penguin. Read by Heather Bell.

The House in Paris by Elizabeth Bowen, published by Chivers/Penguin. Read by Sian Thomas.

Kidnapped by Robert Louis Stevenson, various editions. Read by John Samson.

Love for Lydia by H. E. Bates, published by Michael Joseph/Penguin. Read by Roy Spencer.

A Month in the Country by J. L. Carr, published by Harvester/Penguin. Read by Nigel Hawthorne.

More Work for the Undertaker by Margery Allingham, published by

Heinemann. Read by Stephen Murray.

Mrs Miniver by Jan Struther, published by Futura. Read by Faith Brook.

An Open Book by Monica Dickens, published by Heinemann/Penguin. Read by Jennie Goossens.

The Opportunity of a Lifetime by Emma Smith, published by Hamish Hamilton. Read by Penelope Lee.

Pied Piper by Nevil Shute, published by Heinemann/Pan. Read by John Westbrook.

A Portrait of Jane Austen by David Cecil, published by Constable/Penguin. Read by Lockwood West.

The River by Rumer Godden, published by Macmillan. Read by Anne Harvey.

The Sidmouth Letters by Jane Gardam, published by Hamish Hamilton. Read by Prunella Scales.

Skin Deep and Other Stories by Edith Reveley, published by Collins. Read by Margaret Robertson.

A Small Country by Sian James, published by Collins. Read by Sian Phillips.

Smallbone Deceased by Michael Gilbert, published by Hodder and Stoughton. Read by Peter Copley.

The Snow Kitten by Nina Warner Hooke, published by Puffin. Read by Brenda Bruce.

The Spy's Wife by Reginald Hill, published by Penguin. Read by Carole Hayman.

The Temptation of Jack Orkney: Collected Stories, Volume 2 by Doris Lessing, published by Cape. Read by Alec McCowen.

Tolstoy Remembered by Tatyana Tolstoy, published by Michael Joseph. Read by Jill Balcon.

Unreliable Memoirs by Clive James, published by Cape/Picador. Read by the author.

An Unsuitable Job for a Woman by P. D. James, published by Faber/Sphere. Read by Judith Coke.

Up the Crossing by Ken Ausden, published by BBC Publications. Read by Geoffrey Matthews.

With Scarlet Majors by Deborah Morris, published by Hammond and Hammond. Read by Suzanne Delaney.

'Abercrombie's Aunt' by Jan Webster, from *The Punch Book of Short Stories*, published by Penguin. Read by David Allister.

'Angels and Ministers of Grace' and 'Dividends' by Sean O'Faolain, from *Selected Stories of Sean O'Faolain*, published by Constable; 'Childybawn', from *The Stories of Sean O'Faolain*, published by Penguin. Read by T. P. McKenna.

'The Europe That Was' by Geoffrey Household, from *The Europe That Was*, published by David and Charles. Read by Jonathan Newth.